PRECLINICAL DRUG DISPOSITION

DRUGS AND THE PHARMACEUTICAL SCIENCES

A Series of Textbooks and Monographs

Edited by

James Swarbrick
School of Pharmacy
University of North Carolina
Chapel Hill, North Carolina

Additional Volumes in Preparation

PRECLINICAL DRUG DISPOSITION

A Laboratory Handbook

Francis L. S. Tse
James M. Jaffe

Sandoz Research Institute
East Hanover, New Jersey

Marcel Dekker, Inc.   New York • Basel • Hong Kong

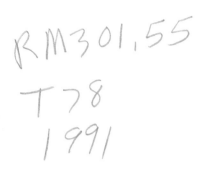
Library of Congress Cataloging-in-Publication Data

Tse, Francis L. S.
    Preclinical drug disposition: a laboratory handbook/Francis
L. S. Tse and James M. Jaffe.
        p.   cm. -- (Drugs and the pharmaceutical sciences; v. 46)
    Includes bibliographical references and index.
    ISBN 0-8247-8500-2 (acid-free paper)
    1. Drugs--Metabolism--Handbooks, manuals, etc.
2. Pharmacokinetics--Handbooks, manuals, etc. 3. Pharmacology,
Experimental--Handbooks, manuals, etc. I. Jaffe, James M.,
    II. Title. III. Title: Pre-clinical drug disposition.
IV. Series.
RM301.55.T78   1991
615 .7--dc20   90-28573
                                                                       CIP

This book is printed on acid-free paper.

MARCEL DEKKER, INC.
270 Madison Avenue, New York, New York 10016

Current printing (last digit):
10 9 8 7 6 5 4 3 2 1

PRINTED IN THE UNITED STATES OF AMERICA

To Irene and Clara

and

To Judy, Tracey, Julie, and Millie

Preface

We have been concerned for some time with the lack of a laboratory manual pertaining specifically to the conduct of drug disposition studies. These types of studies normally define the absorption, distribution, metabolism, and excretion (ADME) of test compounds in animals and humans. Such information is vital to the proper understanding of the pharmacological and toxicological properties associated with the compound. While there is an abundance of reference books on the theoretical aspects of drug absorption, disposition, and pharmacokinetics, no comprehensive text is currently available concerning the practical details of experimental procedures and data interpretation necessary for these studies.

During the past ten years, we have been involved with a preclinical research group that primarily is responsible for the pharmacokinetic investigation of new drug candidates in animals. In order to comply with regulatory requirements, i.e., good laboratory practices (GLPs), it was necessary to develop a great number of standard operating procedures (SOPs) describing the experimental methods used in our laboratory for conducting drug disposition studies. This handbook summarizes some of the more basic, in vivo procedures so that they can be shared by others. In vitro and in situ techniques (e.g., protein binding, everted intestinal sac, organ perfusion) designed specifically to explore the underlying principles of drug disposition have been intentionally omitted. Additionally, the less commonly employed species (e.g., hamsters, guinea pigs, mini-pigs) and routes of drug administration (e.g., rectal, nasal, topical) are not addressed.

The book focuses on the practical aspects of the conduct of drug disposition studies in common laboratory animals. Chapter 1 presents the fundamental concepts of ADME and the general objectives of nonclinical pharmacokinetic studies. Chapter 2 describes the use of radioactivity in drug disposition studies. Radioactive tracers provide a simple means of monitoring the administered dose in the body and are particularly important during the early stages of drug development when specific analytical methods are often unavailable. Chapters 3-7 concern specific details of experimental procedures in commonly used laboratory species, i.e., rat, mouse, dog, rabbit, and monkey, respectively. The discussions focus on the types of experiments, study design, animal preparation and maintenance, dose administration, and biological sample collection and preparation for analysis. Chapter 8 is devoted to the proper interpretation of results using established pharmacokinetic methods. Because of differences in experimental conditions and design between animal and human ADME studies, the approach used in evaluating the data also can vary.

We hope this text will be useful as a primary source of information to researchers in universities, chemical and pharmaceutical concerns, and regulatory agencies. It should also serve as a basic reference for undergraduate and graduate students preparing for a research career in drug metabolism and pharmacokinetics.

We are grateful to our colleagues in the Pharmacokinetics Section of Sandoz Research Institute for their valuable contributions to the development and maintenance of the SOPs that form the foundation of this text: R. Aun, F. Ballard, W. Caubet, T. Chang, S. Elmansoury, C. Farley, D. Galluccio, D. Guthardt, B. Juranich, K. Marty, J. Minish, D. Nickerson, B. Paterson, and J. Skinn. We are also indebted to Rosemary Valentino and Lisa Olbis for their assistance in the preparation of the manuscript.

Francis L. S. Tse
James M. Jaffe

Contents

PRECLINICAL DRUG DISPOSITION

1

Introduction

Fundamental Concepts of ADME

In a broad sense, disposition includes all processes and factors that are involved from the time a drug is administered to the time it is eliminated from the body, either in the unchanged form or as a biotransformation product (metabolite). More specifically, the term encompasses the processes of *absorption*, *distribution*, *metabolism*, and *excretion* (ADME), which are depicted in Fig. 1.1.

Absorption

Absorption is the process by which a test compound and its metabolites are transferred from the site of absorption to the systemic circulation. In animal disposition studies, the test compound is most commonly administered orally – either by gavage (intubation) as a solid (e.g., capsule); as a liquid dosage form (e.g., solution, suspension); or, often in rodents, as a drug-food mixture (dietary admixture). In either case, as illustrated in Fig. 1.1, the rate of absorption can be markedly influenced by how rapidly the test material dissolves in the gas-

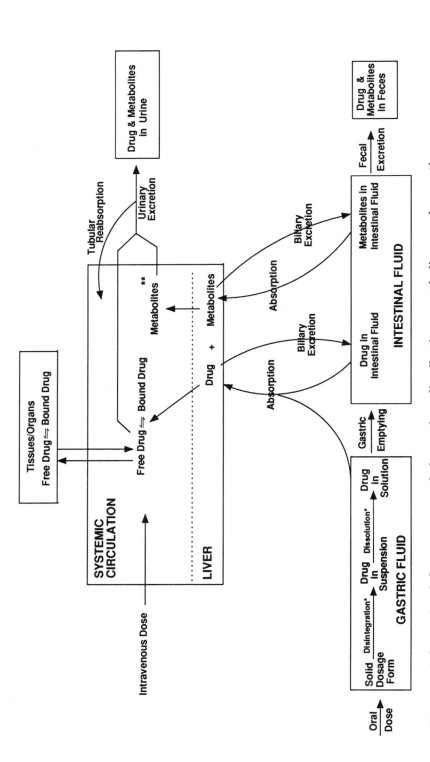

FIG. 1.1 Schematic of the processes of absorption, distribution, metabolism, and excretion.

*Processes that can occur in the intestinal tract.

**Similar to the drug, metabolites can be bound or free, and the free metabolite can be distributed to the tissues/organs.

trointestinal fluids. This is referred to as the dissolution process and is often the rate-limiting step in the absorption process that can subsequently influence the onset, duration, and intensity of the pharmacological activity of the test substance. For this reason, absorption is usually most rapid and less variable for a solution as compared to a solid dosage form, especially for relatively water-insoluble compounds. Thus various factors that influence solubility such as particle size, salt form, pH, crystalline structure, and solvent systems play an important role in modifying the absorption process and must be considered in designing animal experiments.

In addition to solubility, other physicochemical factors can also influence the absorption of a drug solution in the gastrointestinal tract. These include instability as a result of digestive enzymes or low gastric pH, and drug complexation due to the presence of dietary components. Other factors such as presystemic metabolism, either in the gut wall or the liver (first-pass effect), which often affect the systemic availability of the parent compound (bioavailability), have relatively minor effects on the total absorption (exposure) of drug and related materials.

In the absence of the above effects, once a compound is in a form (solution) in the gastrointestinal tract that can be absorbed, it will then pass through the gastrointestinal mucosa, a semipermeable membrane, into the blood, normally by a process referred to as passive diffusion. Three factors – the pKa and the lipid solubility of the compound and the pH at the absorption site – will govern its movement through the membrane in this manner. The influence of these is collectively referred to as the pH-partition hypothesis. Thus the nonionized form of an acidic or basic drug will be preferentially absorbed by diffusion, with the driving force for movement through the membrane being the concentration gradient (i.e., the difference between the concentration of solute in the gastrointestinal tract and that in the blood). The greater the proportion of drug in the nonionized to ionized form at the absorption site, the more rapid and efficient the absorption process. Acidic compounds will usually be absorbed from the stomach while basic drugs will be absorbed from the more alkaline milieu of the intestines. Additionally, the rate and extent of absorption are related to the oil/water partition coefficient so that the more lipophilic the compound, the more rapid and efficient is its absorption.

Although most compounds cross the intestinal membrane by a diffusion mechanism, many natural substances such as vitamins and l-amino acids as well as some drugs are absorbed by a structurally specific active transport process in which molecules move from the mucosal to the serosal side of the gastrointestinal tract regardless of the concentration gradient. This is an enzymatic process which can be saturated at high drug concentrations and has the potential for competitive inhibition if two similar substrates are transported by the same carrier mechanism. Also, since the active transport process consumes energy, it can be inhibited by substances that interfere with cell metabolism. Although other absorption mechanisms such as facilitated diffusion, pinocytosis, convective absorption, ion-pair absorption, and lymphatic absorption have been identified and can also be important, they are responsible for the transport of relatively few compounds.

Distribution

After entering the bloodstream, the molecules of the compound mix with body fluids and are then distributed to the site of action. Initially, the highly perfused organs (heart, liver, kidney) receive the majority of the dose with delivery of the compound to organs such as muscle, skin, and fat much more slowly. The differences between organs in lipophilicity, blood supply, and ability to interact with foreign substances make drug concentrations nonuniform throughout the body. Thus the distribution of a compound can have a profound effect on the onset, intensity, and duration of pharmacological response.

The distribution of compounds in the blood into its various components (red cells, white cells, plasma proteins, plasma water) is important since only the free drug (see Fig. 1.1) distributes to body tissues. Due to specific binding, for example to plasma proteins, hemoglobin, and blood cell walls, there can be substantial differences between circulating whole blood and plasma concentrations of the administered compound. Thus it is critical to clearly define the type of biological sample utilized for analysis.

The main interaction in the blood is the binding to various plasma proteins, mainly albumin for acidic drugs and α_1-acid glycoprotein for basic compounds. Most binding is by reversible physical forces, and stronger (covalent) binding is rare. Also, since the binding site on acids is usually the N-terminal amino acid while bases appear to bind nonspecifically, the capacity of protein binding to acids is limited while that of binding to bases is usually large. In general, only when the percent binding is high ($>95\%$) will the plasma serve as a significant storage compartment for compounds.

Outside the blood compartment, molecules that are not bound (free molecules) in the blood and do not have molecular weights of > 500-600 can penetrate the capillary walls and reach the interstitial spaces. An essentially protein-free ultrafiltrate fluid of plasma carries nonprotein-bound materials in either direction across the capillary walls by hydrostatic pressure.

The membranes of the tissues behave in a similar manner to those of the gastrointestinal tract; i.e., lipid soluble, nonprotein-bound molecules pass through the membranes by a passive diffusion process where equilibrium is established between the inside and outside of the tissue. Thus, for most compounds, penetration depends on a favorable un-ionized to ionized ratio. For example lipid-soluble compounds with molecular weights of < 1000 can cross the placental barrier by simple diffusion while the membrane is essentially impregnable to highly polar material. The extent of tissue localization in any particular tissue is related to the physicochemical property of the compound as well as to the ratio of plasma-to-tissue concentration. The rate of tissue localization, though, is mainly dependent on the blood flow to that area. Thus equilibrium occurs rather rapidly in the highly perfused organs such as the kidney and lung, relatively more slowly in moderately perfused muscle tissue and skin, and much more slowly in fat. Like other equilibration processes, tissue localization is usually reversible.

The brain capillaries are surrounded by a cellular sheath that makes them substantially less permeable to water-soluble materials than capillaries found in other areas of the body. This is often referred to as the "blood-brain barrier." Thus, the ability of compounds to penetrate areas of the central nervous system (CNS) such as the brain, as well as the cerebrospinal fluid (CSF), is highly dependent on their lipid solubility (o/w partition coefficient). Compounds with more polar characteristics will show little pharmacological activity in these areas.

Metabolism   Metabolism (biotransformation) is the process by which the administered compound is structurally and/or chemically changed in the body by either enzymatic or nonenzymatic reactions. The pathways by which this occurs are classified as either phase I or phase II reactions. Phase I processes convert the compound by oxidation, reduction, or hydrolysis while phase II, often termed conjugation reactions, involves coupling between the compound or its metabolite and endogenous substrate, especially glucuronic or sulfuric acid. Although these reactions can take place in various tissues and organs throughout the body, compounds are predominantly metabolized in the liver by microsomal enzymes located in the endoplasmic reticulum. Normally, metabolism results in a molecule that is substantially less active than the parent compound, although in some phase I reactions, the metabolite may be more active than the parent molecule (prodrug). Also, since metabolites are generally more polar than the original compound, their volumes of distribution are reduced and their ability to be eliminated via the kidneys is greatly increased.

The rate of metabolic enzymatic reactions can usually be described by the Michaelis-Menton equation:

$$\text{Metabolic Rate} = \frac{V_{max} \, C}{K_m + C}$$

where

V_{max} = the maximum production rate of metabolite

C   = the concentration of compound in the blood

K_m = the Michaelis constant

Normally, blood concentrations are much smaller than the K_m values associated with their metabolism and the above equation can be written as:

$$\text{Metabolic Rate} = \frac{V_{max} \, C}{K_m} = k_m \, C$$

where k_m is a first-order metabolic rate constant and, thus, the rate of metabolism is proportional to the blood concentration. At elevated concentrations exceeding the saturation level, the rate of metabolism become nonlinear. Thus, the Michaelis-Menten nature of drug metabolism will result in a decrease in the rate of elimination of compounds at higher dose levels (dose-dependent elimination).

The rate of metabolism can also be decreased due to inhibition of the microsomal enzymes (enzyme inhibition), which can be of a competitive or noncompetitive nature. Competitive inhibition can occur when structurally similar compounds compete for the same site on the enzyme. In noncompetitive inhibition, a substrate of unrelated structure to the compound undergoing metabolism combines with the enzyme to prevent the formation of an enzyme:compound complex.

An increase (stimulation) in the activity of the microsomal enzymes (enzyme induction) can occur by the administration of certain drugs or by exposure to some chemicals in the environment. For example, barbiturates induce the synthesis of cytochrome P-450 and cytochrome P-450 reductase, which increases enzyme activity leading to a corresponding increase in metabolism of a wide variety of structurally unrelated compounds.

Excretion

Compounds are eliminated from the body as the unchanged molecule or as metabolite(s). As stated previously, in most excretory organs except the lungs, water soluble (polar) substances are excreted more efficiently than those that are relatively lipoidal. Although excretion can take place through numerous pathways such as the bile, feces, milk, saliva, perspiration, tears, and lungs, the most significant organ for elimination is the kidney. Renal excretion involves three processes:

1. Passive glomerular filtration
2. Active tubular secretion
3. Passive tubular reabsorption

The amount of material entering the tubular lumen by filtration is dependent on the filtration rate and the degree of plasma-protein binding. Active tubular secretion occurs in the proximal renal tubule and involves the carrier-mediated transfer of anions or cations from the renal interstitial fluid to the tubular fluid. Weak organic acid and bases are usually involved in this process. In the proximal and distal tubules passive reabsorption of compounds from the glomerular filtrate back into the blood (see Fig. 1.1) is influenced by the intrinsic lipid solubility of the compound, its ionization constant, and the pH of the urine. Thus, compounds of high lipid solubility do not appear in the urine in large proportions because most of the molecules filtered at the glomerulus return to blood by diffusing across the lipidlike boundary of the tubular cells. Conversely, compounds of low lipid solubility are readily excreted in the urine because they are poorly reabsorbed in the tubule. Because of this, the pH of the tubular fluid and the dissociation constant of the compound being excreted often influence the renal tubular transfer of many weak acids and bases, just as these same factors influence the absorption of compounds in the gastrointestinal tract as discussed previously.

Hepatic elimination can also play an important role in the excretion process. Compounds that are metabolized in the liver are often excreted in the bile into the intestinal tract (see Fig. 1.1). Here they can be reabsorbed by passive diffusion into the blood (enterohepatic recycling) or excreted in the feces along with unabsorbed material following oral administration. Factors such as molecular weight, chemical structure, polarity, species, sex, and the nature of the metabolic process affect the rate and extent of biliary elimination. Both organic anions, including glucuronides, and organic cations are actively transported into bile by carrier mechanisms similar to those described for transport of substances across gastrointestinal and renal membranes.

Excretion by other routes (perspiration, saliva, tears, milk) is quantitatively insignificant in relation to urine and feces (bile). Mammary excretion though can be of potential importance for highly potent compounds that could induce toxic manifestations in the nursing newborn whose hepatic and renal detoxification capacity are usually limited.

Objectives of Nonclinical ADME Studies

Support for
Pharmacol-
ogy

It is well recognized that the intensity and duration of the pharmacologic effect of a systemically
acting drug are functions, not only of the intrinsic
activity of the drug, but also of its absorption, distribution, and elimination characteristics. ADME
data obtained from the pharmacologic test species
are often useful in the interpretation of drug effects, such as in the case where a drug is active
following intravenous administration but is considerably less active after oral dosing. Appropriate
ADME data can indicate whether the drug is poorly
absorbed, resulting in subtherapeutic blood levels,
or undergoes presystemic biotransformation to
an inactive metabolite. This provides information
for subsequent decisions such as improving drug
absorption by alteration in the salt form or formulation, investigation of the possibility of prodrugs,
or abandonment of the oral route of administration.

Knowledge of the pharmacologically efficacious
systemic concentration in animal models can be
utilized to guide later studies in humans. During
the initial, clinical efficacy trials, doses should be
escalated at least until plasma concentrations comparable to those resulting from an active dose in
the pharmacologic species are achieved. In the
absence of adverse effects (toxicity), a drug should
not be considered ineffective if only subtherapeutic drug concentrations are attained.

Support for
Toxicology

Probably the most important function of animal
ADME studies is in support of nonclinical drug-
safety evaluation (animal toxicity trials) Generally, in subchronic toxicology studies, the drug is

administered orally to the test species, often with no assurance of absorption or dose proportionality. Since the absorption (exposure) is a critical parameter in the validation of toxicology studies, both from a scientific and regulatory perspective, this factor must be addressed for each animal model as well as for the specific mode of administration.

Determination of ADME characteristics during the course of toxicology study may also aid in the interpretation of certain toxicologic findings. For example, tissue distribution data may be useful in explaining organ specific toxic manifestations. The occurence of enzyme inhibition or capacity-limited metabolism may result in drug accumulation accompanied by toxicity.

Comparison of the ADME data obtained from animals with those from man may provide a rational selection of an appropriate animal model for long-term toxicity testing, e.g., carcinogenicity and teratogenicity studies that will give a reliable prediction of human safety. Qualitative similarities in the overall metabolite patterns between the test species and man ensure that both are exposed to the same compounds (drug and metabolites). Additionally, it is desirable that the laboratory animal demonstrates similar absorption and excretion characteristics as humans.

Prediction of Human ADME

Preclinical data on drug absorption and disposition can support and guide informed decisions concerning initial trials in humans during a period when minimal clinical information regarding the drug is available. Animal data may also be helpful in the design of human ADME studies. For many drugs, the extent of absorption is very consistent between different animal species and man.

The actual form of the drug reaching the systemic circulation, however, may differ among species due to the large qualitative and quantitative differences in the metabolism of a drug among species. Thus, interspecies variations in such important pharmacokinetic parameters as absolute bioavailability, clearance, and elimination half-life will occur for the same compound preventing a valid, direct extrapolation of animal disposition data to man. In this situation human pharmacokinetic characteristics can be estimated by "interspecies scaling," which is based on similarities in anatomy, physiology, and biochemistry among animal models and man. Unfortunately, this approach normally requires at least three to four animal species to properly make a valid prediction. Such information is often unavailable during the preclinical phase which, ironically, is also the time when an accurate prediction of human response to the drug would be most useful.

Development of New Dosage Forms and Formulations

Animal models are often employed to provide support in the development of new dosage forms or formulations. Initially, ADME studies describe the disposition characteristics of the drug and can serve as the basis for the selection of a suitable dosage form. For example, specific information on the site of absorption can be obtained from laboratory animals by simple surgery that would be difficult and unethical to perform in man. This knowledge can be used to determine the need for such specific dosage forms as enteric-coated or controlled-release units. Additionally, animals are often used as a screen for new dosage forms in order to eliminate unnecessary human trials with formulations having potentially suboptimal in vivo performance.

These studies can reduce the cost and time necessary for developing a new form or formulation as well as avoid unnecessary human exposure to test compounds. Thus, formulations with desirable in vitro release patterns as demonstrated by dissolution profiles would be submitted for definitive bioavailability testing in humans only if they first demonstrated the desired blood-level profile in an animal model.

The key to successful use of animal data in this manner is the selection of a proper model. While there is limited information concerning direct comparisons of drug absorption in humans and laboratory animals, the beagle dog has proved to be the most commonly used animal species in bioavailability studies. Oral dosage forms intended for humans generally can be administered intact to dogs. Dogs are relatively easy to maintain and handle and their body weight is stable over time to allow repeated studies in the same animal (crossover designs). A 10-kg dog allows for at least 10 relatively large serial blood samples (3 ml/time point) to be obtained over the course of 24 hours and for repeated studies at one to two week intervals. Additionally, dog and man share many similarities in gastrointestinal anatomy and physiology and, although the dog may differ from man in the absolute bioavailability of drugs due to possible differences in first-pass metabolism, it appears to be a good indicator of the relative bioavailability of different dosage forms or formulations.

2

Use of Radioactivity in Drug Disposition Studies

The rapid growth of knowledge in the field of drug metabolism and disposition reflects to a large extent the utilization of radioactive isotopes as tracers of chemical and biological processes. Appropriately radiolabeled test compounds are often used in ADME studies, since this method provides a simple means of monitoring the administered dose in the body. This is particularly important during the early stage of drug development when specific analytical methods are often unavailable. The use of total radioactivity measurements allows an estimation of the total exposure to drug-related material and facilitates the achievement of material balance.

Commonly Used Radio-nuclides

The most commonly used radionuclides in drug metabolism and disposition studies are carbon-14 (^{14}C) and tritium (^{3}H), both of which are referred to as beta, or negatron, emitters. Since these beta-emitting isotopes have relatively long half-lives (see Table 2.1), their radioactive decay during an experiment is insignificant. Additionally, they provide sufficient emission energy for measurement and are relatively safe to use, as indicated by the data in Table 2.1. Although any individual beta particle can have any energy up to the maximum, E_{max}, the basic quantity in determining the energy imparted to tissues by beta emitters is the average energy, $\dot{E}_\beta$. The range is the maximum thickness the beta particles can penetrate. For example, the beta particles from tritium are stopped by only 6 mm of air or about 5 μm of water, and present virtually no hazard when they originate outside the body (1).

Biologic Stability

During the synthesis of radiolabeled compounds, the label is usually introduced as part of the molecular skeleton and specifically into a metabolically stable and, in the case of tritium, nonexchange-

TABLE 2.1 Some Properties of Tritium and Carbon-14

Property	^{3}H	^{14}C
Half-life (yr)	12.3	5730
Maximum beta energy (MeV)	0.0186	0.156
Average beta energy (MeV)	0.006	0.049
Range in air (mm)	6	300
Range in unit density material (mm)	0.0052	0.29

Source: Data from Ref. 1.

able position. The in vivo stability of ^{14}C labels is often reflected by the extent of [^{14}C] carbon dioxide formation, which will be discussed in association with the topic of excretion in later chapters. The biologic stability of ^{3}H labels can be estimated by the extent of tritiated water formation. The tritiated water concentration (dpm/ml) in the distillate or lyophylisate of urine samples collected during a designated time interval after dosing, presumably after equilibrium is reached between urine and the body water pool, is determined. This value is extrapolated from the midpoint of the collection interval to zero time, based on the known half-life of tritiated water in the given species. The percentage of the radioactive dose that is transformed to tritiated water ($\%^{3}H_2O$) can be calculated using the following equation:

$$\%^{3}H_2O \doteq \frac{\begin{array}{c}{}^{3}H_2O \\ \text{concentration} \\ \text{at zero time}\end{array} \times \begin{array}{c}\text{exchangeable} \\ \text{body water} \\ \text{volume}\end{array}}{\text{radioactivity dose}} \times 100\%$$

Values for the exchangeable body water content as well as the half-life of tritiated water in some mammalian species that can be applied to the above equation are shown in Table 2.2 (2,3). If the drug is likely to or is known to fragment into two major portions, it may be desirable to monitor both fragments by providing each with a different tracer (^{3}H and ^{14}C).

Purity and Specific Activity

The chemical and radiochemical purity of the labeled compound must be ascertained prior to use. Absolute radiochemical purity is difficult to attain so that in practice a value of $\geq 95\%$ is usually acceptable. The desired specific activity of the

TABLE 2.2 Volume and Half-Life of Body Water in Some Mammalian Species

Species	Sex	Exchangeable body water (% of body weight)	Half-life (days)
Mouse	F	58.5	1.13
Rat	M	59.6	3.53
Rabbit	F	58.4	3.87
Dog	M	66.0	5.14
Cynomolgus monkey	F	64.2	7.23
Rhesus monkey	M	61.6	7.80
Man	M, F	55.3	9.46

Source: Data from Refs. 2 and 3.

administered radioactive compound depends on the dose to be used as well as the species studied. A logical approach is to use minimal radioactivity that allows the description of the time course of the labeled substance in the animal for a sufficient period of time. Doses of ^{14}C of the order of 5 μCi/kg for the dog and 20 μCi/kg for the rat have been found adequate in most ADME studies, while doses of ^{3}H are usually two to three times higher owing to lower counting efficiency of this isotope.

Liquid Scintillation Counting

Liquid scintillation counting is the most popular technique for the detection and measurement of radioactivity. In order to count a liquid specimen such as plasma, urine, or digested blood or tissues directly in a liquid-scintillation spectrometer, an aliquot of the specimen is first mixed with a liquid scintillant. Aliquots of blood, feces, or tissue homogenates are air-dried on ash-free filter papers and combusted in a sample oxidizer provided with an appropriate absorption medium and a liquid scintillant prior to counting. The liquid scintillant plays the role of an energy transducer, converting energy from nuclear decay into light. The light generates electrical signal pulses which are analyzed according to their timing and amplitude, and are subsequently recorded as a count rate, e.g., counts per minute (cpm). Based on the counting efficiency of the radionuclide used, the count rate is then converted to the rate of disintegration, e.g., disintegrations per minute (dpm), which is a representation of the amount of radioactivity present in the sample.

Further work on these samples utilizing specific techniques such as high-pressure liquid chromatography coupled with radioactivity monitoring (HPLC/RAM) or reverse isotope dilution (HPLC/RID) allows the determination of the components of this mixture (drug and/or metabolites). Although not within the scope of this book, conventional analytical methods including gas chromatography, liquid chromatography, radioimmunoassay, fluorometry, etc., certainly can be applied to determine the concentration of the parent compound and known metabolites in both radioactive and nonradioactive samples.

Statistics of Liquid Scintillation Counting

It should be noted that radioactive disintegrations are a random process. Therefore, the true count rate is more accurately determined if a greater number of counts are accumulated over a longer

period of counting time. For most counting pur-
poses, it is adequate to count to a "2 sigma (σ) percent error" which involves a confidence level of
95%. This means that subsequent measurements
will fall within the 2σ error 95 times out of 100.
The basic 2σ error is:

$$\frac{2\sqrt{N}}{N} \times 100\%$$

where N represents the total count (4). A list of 2σ
errors is given in Table 2.3. In order to obtain the
same degree of accuracy in analyzing different
samples in any given study, all samples should be
counted to the same statistical error, i.e., until
the same number of total counts is accumulated.
This counting strategy contrasts the common, although incorrect, practice of counting all samples for a preset time period regardless of their
radioactivity level. In relatively new liquid scintillation spectrometer models, however, the user
can control the system so that counting is terminated when the selected statistical error value
or time terminator is reached, whichever occurs
first. The time terminator in this case is set only
to prevent excessive counting of samples with very
low radioactivity levels such as blank samples.

The selection of an acceptable statistical error requires a somewhat arbitrary decision. A useful
rule is that samples need not be counted to a percent error smaller than the maximum experimental error accrued during sample preparation,
for the final calculations which include the count
rates cannot be more precise than the maximum
experimental error. Maximum experimental error

TABLE 2.3 Counting Errors at 95% Confidence
Level from Different Total Counts Accumulated

Total counts accumulated	2σ error (95% confidence level)	
	Percentage	Counts
1,000,000	0.2	2,000
444,444	0.3	1,333
160,000	0.5	800
81,632	0.7	571
40,000	1.0	400
17,777	1.5	267
10,000	2.0	200
4,444	3.0	133
1,600	5.0	80
816	7.0	57
400	10.0	40
177	15.0	27
100	20.0	20

Source: Data from Ref. 4.

includes all errors that arise during the processes
of dosing, sample collection, pipetting, weighing,
analysis, and other related laboratory procedures.

Sensitivity of Liquid Scintillation Counting

The limit of sensitivity of liquid scintillation counting can be determined based on the "uncertainty
of a difference" statistic. In radioactivity measurements, the sample count rate (net cpm) is obtained

by subtracting a background (background cpm) from the gross count rate (gross cpm). Thus, the error or uncertainty in net cpm (U_n) arises from the errors in both background cpm (U_b) and gross cpm (U_g) as follows:

$$U_n = \sqrt{(U_b)^2 + (U_g)^2}$$

where U_b and U_g at 2σ confidence are calculated from the respective total count, N, and the counting time, t, as

$$2 \times \sqrt{\frac{N}{t^2}}$$

The following example illustrates the calculation of the sensitivity limit using the above equations.

Example 1

A sample has a gross cpm of 27. The background cpm is 25. Accepting a 2σ error of $\pm 7\%$, counting is terminated after reaching 816 counts (see Table 2.3), i.e., after counting the sample for 816/27 or 30.22 min and the background vial for 816/25 or 32.64 min.

$$U_b = 2 \times \sqrt{\frac{816}{(32.64)^2}}$$

$$= 1.75$$

$$U_g = 2 \times \sqrt{\frac{816}{(30.22)^2}}$$

$$= 1.89$$

$$U_n = \sqrt{(1.75)^2 + (1.89)^2}$$
$$= 2.58$$

Thus, net cpm $= (27 - 25) \pm 2.58$
$$= 2 \pm 2.58$$

Since the 95% confidence interval $(-0.58 - 4.58)$ includes zero, it can be deduced that a net cpm ≤ 2 is not significantly different from zero. Using the same procedure, it can also be shown that any net count ≥ 3 cpm is detectable.

Although the minimum detectable net count rate is 3 cpm in the above example, the degree of uncertainty or error associated with it is relatively large. The error percentage decreases with increasing count rate, as shown in Table 2.4. Hence the

TABLE 2.4 Errors at 95% Confidence Level Associated with Different Net Count Rates, Assuming a Background of 25 cpm[a]

Gross cpm	Net cpm	Error percentage of net cpm
28	3 ± 2.63	87.7
30	5 ± 2.73	54.6
35	10 ± 3.01	30.1
40	15 ± 3.30	22.0
45	20 ± 3.60	18.0
50	25 ± 3.91	15.6
55	30 ± 4.23	14.1
60	35 ± 4.55	13.0
65	40 ± 4.88	12.2

[a]All samples are counted to a 2σ error of $\pm$ 7%.

actual limit of detection should be the lowest count rate which yields an acceptable error level. This could be at a gross cpm of 50 (twice background) in this example, since greater count rates only result in minimal reductions in percent error. It should be noted that the values given in Table 2.4 are calculated based on a mean background of 25 cpm. A greater background count rate would result in a higher limit of detection.

Radiation Protection

Any use of radiolabeled substances requires an understanding of the potential hazards involved. The investigator must be familiar with all related governmental and institutional regulations such as Parts 19 and 20 of Title 10, Chapter 1, *Energy Code of Federal Regulations.* Although most institutions today have radiation safety committees that are specially trained to oversee the proper use of radiation sources, the ultimate responsibility for the safe use of radioactive materials in each laboratory must rest with the authorized user in charge of that laboratory.

Most of the precautions that should be observed when handling the weak beta emitters (^3H and ^{14}C) are similar to those pertaining to any chemical research area where good laboratory practices are applied (5). Some general procedures to be followed in handling radiochemicals are:

1. Segregate radiochemical work from other experiments using nonradiolabeled chemicals, preferably in different rooms.

2. Use minimal quantities of radioactivity.

3. In addition to the normal lab coat, wear thin, latex surgical gloves as a routine practice.

4. Never pipette radioactive liquids by mouth.

5. Always work in a fume hood when using volatile radioactive material.

6. Segregate low- and high-level radioactive materials.

7. Properly label all containers indicating nuclide, compound, total activity/specific activity, date, name of user.

8. Always check "old" material for radiochemical and chemical purity.

9. Always store material as indicated on the product specification sheet.

10. Dispose of radioactive waste according to safety regulations for both solvents and radiation.

11. Entrances to areas where radioactivity is used should be posted with appropriate radioactivity warning signs.

12. In the event of a spill, minimize possible spread of contamination and notify the Radiation Safety Officer immediately.

References

1. J. Shapiro, *Radiation Protection,* 2nd Ed., Harvard University Press, Cambridge, Massachusetts, 1981, pp. 12-18.

2. C. R. Richmond, W. H. Langham, and T. T. Trujillo, Comparative metabolism of tritiated water by mammals, *J. Cell. Comp. Physiol., 59*:45-53, 1962.

3. E. Azar and S. T. Shaw, Jr., Effective body water half-life and total body water in rhesus and cynomolgus monkeys, *Can. J. Physiol. Pharmocol., 53*: 935-939, 1975.

4. E. C. Long, *Liquid Scintillation Counting Theory and Techniques*, Beckman Instruments, Fullerton, California, 1976, p. 36.

5. *Guide for Users of Labelled Compounds*, 3rd Ed., Amersham Corporation, Arlington Heights, Illinois, 1979, p. 20.

3

The Rat

The rat is the most commonly used animal in drug metabolism and disposition studies because it can be easily acquired, is relatively inexpensive, easily housed and handled, and if selected properly has low genetic variability, resulting in a narrower range of response than many other laboratory species. The smaller size of the rat compared with other laboratory species such as the dog and the monkey usually implies the need for a smaller amount of test compound, an important consideration particularly during the early stages of development of the compound. The rat also demonstrates a good survival rate from surgical trauma and, therefore, is frequently used in studies requiring surgical preparations of the animal model. Consequently, a wealth of data on the anatomy, physiology, and pharmacology of the rat are available for reference.

On the other hand, there are certain disadvantages associated with the small body size of the rat. In general, it is difficult to administer solid-dosage forms (tablets and capsules) to a rat. The size of biological specimens that can be collected is also small compared with larger laboratory animals such as the dog or monkey. Although serial blood sampling from the rat is possible, the volume is limited to about 200 μl at collection intervals typical of a pharmacokinetic study. Furthermore, rats are not used for multiple experiments due to rapid changes in body weight over a relatively short life span (approx. 2 yr).

Dosing

Oral

In ADME studies oral doses are most commonly given by gastric intubation (gavage) as a solution or a suspension. Solid dosage forms (e.g., tablets, capsules) normally cannot be administered due to the small animal size and, therefore, the difficulty in preparing a correspondingly small dosage form. For chronic administration it is often more convenient to give oral doses incorporated in the diet, although this method has the disadvantage of lacking control over the amount of drug delivered and the time of dose, as well as not mimicking the usual pulse-dose administration used in humans. Since the absorption and metabolism of a drug can be a function of the dosage form, the appropriate oral dosing procedure must be applied to meet the specific objectives of the study.

Gavage

Ideally, the dose is prepared as a solution in a suitable vehicle in order to avoid formulation-related problems in the absorption of the compound. Commonly used solvents include water, ethanol, polyethylene glycol (PEG), propylene glycol, and lipids. Solubility can be enhanced by the use of co-solvents, pH adjustment, or a different crystalline form.

Furthermore, the rate of dissolution can be increased by agitation, heat, and particle-size reduction. The latter can often be accomplished by simple trituration using a mortar and pestle. In those instances when the compound is not entirely soluble at the desired concentration, a suspension is normally prepared. Since the insoluble particles can settle too rapidly for accurate dose measurement, a suspending agent such as methylcellulose or carboxymethylcellulose (CMC) is often incorporated. After preparation it is critical that the suspension be continuously stirred until all animals have been dosed to assure uniform drug administration. Additionally, unless the stability of the liquid preparation has been established, it is advisable that only freshly prepared doses be used.

The liquid doses are given using an animal feeding needle (15-18 G, 3 in) attached to a syringe (Fig. 3.1). A practical dosing volume is approximately 10 ml per kg of body weight. The rat is firmly held by the skin of the neck and back, and is positioned so that the mouth is in line with the esophagus. The needle is passed into the mouth and pushed gently into the stomach until the hub of the needle almost touches the rat's teeth. The drug is then rapidly discharged. Possible obstruction to the needle can occur in two areas, the back of the mouth and at the sphincter to the entrance of the stomach. Misdosing usually results in severe struggling or appearance of the dose preparation in the mouth or nose, indicating that the dose has been given intratracheally (into the lungs). Misdosed animals should be discarded.

Drug-diet mixture   Since a small amount of drug is to be mixed with a comparatively large amount of diluent (pulverized diet), a general method known as geometric dilu-

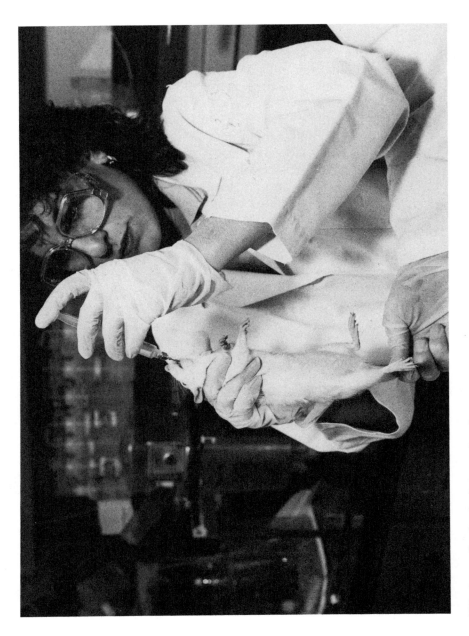

FIG. 3.1   Oral administration by gavage.

tion is usually employed to ensure the uniform distribution of the drug throughout the mixture. In this procedure, the drug is thoroughly triturated with an approximately equal amount of diet using a mortar and pestle. Then a second portion of the pulverized diet equal in amount to the mixture in the mortar is added and the trituration is repeated. This process is continued until all of the diet is incorporated. The above method is suitable for quantities normally used in ADME studies. When larger amounts of the drug-diet mixtures are required, e.g., in long-term safety studies, mechanical mixers such as laboratory scale V-blenders are used. Because of the usually high diet-to-drug ratio in this type of formulation, it is particularly important that content uniformity be confirmed prior to the study.

The drug-diet ratio is determined by the intended dose, the rat weight, and the average daily food consumption, which is approximately 20 g for a 250 g rat. Since the addition of the test compound can alter the taste of the diet, thereby influencing the amount of diet and drug consumed, it is recommended that a pilot test be conducted prior to the actual study. The former will establish an accurate feeding pattern for the particular drug-diet mixture. In cases where food consumption is drastically reduced so that the desired dose cannot be properly administered, small amounts of lactose (1-2%) can be incorporated to enhance palatability. This material is known to be inert and would have no effect on the disposition of the test compound.

The design of the rat cage should be such that any spillage of the mixture can be recovered and will not contaminate the excreta. Certain commercially available models such as the Nalgene® Metabolic Cage described on p. 58 (Collection of Excreta) appear to be well suited for this purpose.

The study is usually conducted over a minimum of 24 hours, which is considered one feeding cycle. Each animal is presented with the estimated daily drug-diet consumption, plus a slight overage which allows for animal variability as well as possible spillage from the rat feeding cup. About 20% overage is adequate for this purpose. The actual dose consumed is recorded at the end of each feeding cycle.

Parenteral

Although parenterally administered drugs may be injected via many routes such as intramuscular, subcutaneous, intrathecal, intracardiac, intraarterial, intraspinal, and intraperitoneal, intravenous dosing is by far the most commonly employed parenteral route in ADME studies. Intravenous administration is not only necessary for testing drugs that are intended for this dose route but also serves as a standard for evaluating the absorption and bioavailability of drugs given via other routes, since intravenous dosing is the only method that eliminates the absorption process by providing direct access to the systemic circulation. In contrast, intraperitoneal administration is not recommended as a reference standard since drug absorption occurs from the peritoneal cavity, is slower, and entails passage into the portal circulation, which can result in incomplete absorption and/or systemic bioavailability.

Intravenous

For intravenous administration, the dose should be prepared as a solution in distilled water or normal saline. If necessary, an appropriate co-solvent such as ethanol or propylene glycol may be used to enhance the solubility of the drug. The practical upper limit of a bolus injection volume is approximately 1 ml per kg body weight. In those cases where solubility problems necessitate larger dose volumes, the dose can be infused over a prolonged period of time. Although it is desirable to consider the pH, isotonicity, and sterility in preparing intravenous solutions, these factors are not critical for a single, acute administration, especially if the volume is not excessive. For example, rats can usually tolerate a fairly wide range of pH, ca. 4.5 to 8, due to the buffering capacity of the blood.

A simple method of intravenous dosing to the rat is by direct injection via the jugular vein exposed surgically under light ether anesthesia (Fig. 3.2). The rat is placed in a closed container such as a covered jar or cage containing cotton or gauze moistened with ether. Following anesthesia, the rat is removed from the container and placed on its back. To maintain anesthesia during the dosing process, the nose of the animal is partially inserted into the opening of a small wide-mouth bottle containing ether-wetted cotton or gauze. This should be sufficient to maintain adequate anesthesia for about 10 min. A small incision is made in the neck of the unconscious rat on one side of midline to expose the jugular vein. In older rats fat and connective tissue can obscure the vein and therefore should be carefully removed. If constriction of the vein occurs as a result of manipulation, it will regain its original size if left undisturbed for approximately 1 to 2 min.

A 25 G needle is inserted at an angle of about 10° through the pectoral muscle (located above the vein) and into the jugular vein, pointing toward the

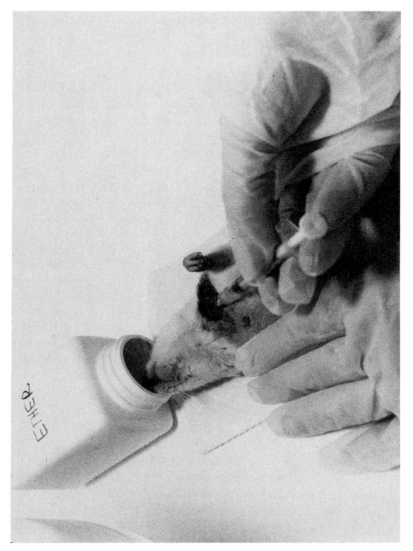

FIG. 3.2 Intravenous injection via the surgically exposed jugular vein.

head of the animal. Following withdrawal of a small volume of blood into the syringe barrel to confirm that the needle is in the vein, the drug solution is injected as quickly as feasible. Passage of the needle through the pectoral muscle is important since the latter acts as a seal and prevents bleeding when the needle is withdrawn. After dosing, the ether chamber is removed from the rat, and the incision is quickly closed with wound clips or sutures.

Although administration via the jugular vein requires surgical preparation of the rat, it appears to be one of the more reliable procedures for intravenous dosing and, unlike most cannulation techniques, imposes no stress, which may affect at least some aspects of normal physiology resulting in altered drug disposition kinetics.

An alternative method of intravenous administration is by injection into the caudal (tail) vein. Although this procedure is relatively simple, involving no surgery and anesthesia, it may not be appropriate if the same vein is also to be used for serial blood collection. Dosing via the caudal vein can result in residual drug at or near the injection site so that sampling from the same location could lead to spurious drug concentrations. Due to the simplicity of this method, though, it is often used for experiments employing a relatively large number of rats designated for exsanguinated blood and tissue collection. The rat is placed in a suitable rodent restrainer with the tail hanging freely (Fig. 3.3). The tail is immersed in a beaker of warm water for 1 to 2 min to dilate the vein and then quickly dried with a towel. The use of a simple desk lamp with a 60-W bulb supplies sufficient heat to keep the vein dilated. A 22 to 25 G needle

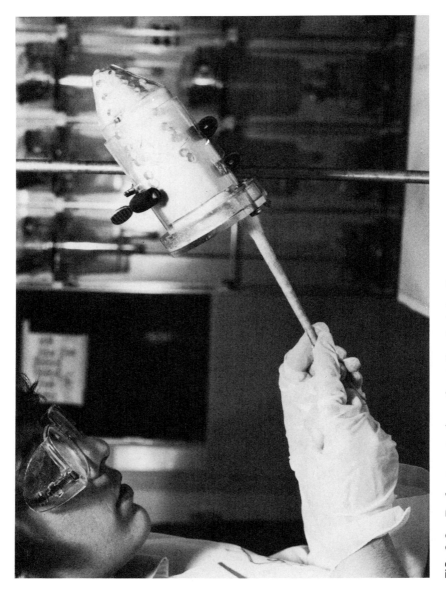

FIG. 3.3 Rodent restrainer for tail-vein injection.

is inserted at an angle of about 10° into one of the two veins. Care should be taken to distinguish the veins (the lateral blood vessels) from the artery which is located at the top center of the tail. After confirming that the needle is in the vein as described previously, the drug solution is injected at a rate of approximately 1 ml/min.

Other veins that have been described for drug administration in the rat include the sublingual, penile, femoral, and dorsal metatarsal veins. Although some of these, e.g., the sublingual vein (1) appear to be suitable, they have not been widely used in ADME studies.

Since rapid intravenous administration of drugs normally results in substantially higher blood levels than oral dosing, tolerance to the test material should be established in a pilot study using 1 to 2 animals. This pretest, using nonradiolabeled drug, is particularly important for experiments involving radiotracers so that the use of radioactivity in the laboratory is minimized.

Intraportal In contrast to other intravenous routes, the portal vein is only used in specific studies, particularly to evaluate the first-pass metabolism of drugs. Unlike the intravenous routes described above, the portal blood flow directly enters the liver prior to reaching the systemic circulation. Comparison of blood-level data obtained from portal vein administration with those after oral and intravenous dosing would indicate the degree of drug absorption and bioavailability, respectively.

The rat is kept under ether anesthesia during the entire procedure. An area on the ventral side is shaved so that a 3 to 4 cm midline incision can be made downward from the sternum. A loop of small intestine containing the bile duct is exteriorized to expose the portal vein. This segment should be kept moist with physiological saline throughout the procedure. For intraportal administration, the dose is injected into one of the tributaries of the portal vein such as the pancreatic, duodenal, mesenteric, or splenic vein through a 27 G needle (Fig. 3.4). Direct injection into the portal vein should be avoided since this often results in excessive blood loss which could also affect the accuracy of the dose. Following injection, a gauze pad is gently pressed on the injection site immediately after removal of the needle. Pressure should

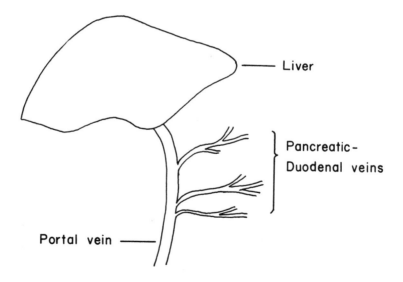

FIG. 3.4 Portal vein and tributary veins in the rat. (Adapted from Ref. 2, with permission of *J. Appl. Physiol.*)

be maintained on the site for approximately 30 sec. The use of a small amount of purified bovine thrombin powder (Pentex®) facilitates rapid clotting. Alternatively, bleeding can be stopped by two ligatures made in the immediate area at the site of puncture. The gut segment is then gently replaced into the body cavity. The incision is closed using silk suture for the muscle layer and suture or wound clips for the skin.

Intra-muscular

Although intramuscular injection does not always provide complete drug delivery to the systemic circulation, it is generally less hazardous than the intravenous route and is particularly useful for administering suspensions or oleaginous solutions which are not suitable for intravenous injection. Drug absorption by this route often is slow and prolonged. The dose is usually injected into the skeletal muscles of the hind limbs, i.e., the biceps femoris, the semitendinosus, or gluteus maximus. The needle should be inserted deeply enough so that its tip is not felt through the skin but should not come into contact with the bone. The size of the needle depends on the viscosity of the vehicle, 25 G being normally employed for aqueous solutions and 21 to 23 G for suspensions or oleaginous solutions. The injection volume is usually 0.1 to 0.2 ml.

Subcuta-neous

Many compounds are routinely given by subcutaneous injection, in particular insulin, local anesthetics, and vaccines. However, this site is not commonly used in ADME studies in animals due to the possibility of causing severe pain, local necrosis, or sterile abscesses. The rate of drug absorption from the subcutaneous injection site rela-

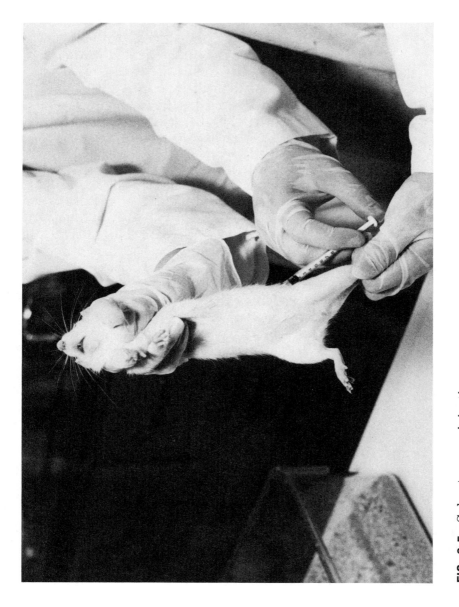

FIG. 3.5 Subcutaneous injection.

tive to intramuscular sites is dependent on the drug as well as the vehicle, although absorption from both routes is usually slower than after intravenous dosing. For subcutaneous injection, the needle should be passed through the skin into the loose interstitial tissues of the side or abdomen, at a shallow angle and pointing toward the head (Fig. 3.5). To minimize leakage of the dose, the needle should be inserted to the hub. Proper placement of the needle can be confirmed by feeling the tip through the skin. The factors governing the needle size used for the subcutaneous route are similar to those described for intramuscular administration although subcutaneous injection volumes can sometimes be greater.

Other parenteral dosage routes
Although other parenteral routes such as intraarterial, intrathecal, and intraspinal dosing have considerable clinical potential for some compounds, they are not well established in nonclinical studies. Intraperitoneal administration is not recommended for ADME studies as previously discussed. Although intracardiac injection appears to yield blood levels similar to those obtained from intravenous doses, the former tends to cause substantial tissue uptake of drug in the heart and should not be used in tissue distribution studies.

Biological Sample Collection

Blood
Since blood (plasma, serum) is the most easily accessible body compartment, the blood concentration profile is most commonly used to describe the time course of drug disposition in the animal.

With the development of sensitive analytical methods that require small volumes (100-200μl) of blood, ADME data from individual rats can be obtained by serial sample collection. Numerous cannulation techniques have been utilized to facilitate repeated blood collection, but the animal preparation procedures are elaborate and tedious and are incompatible with prolonged sampling periods in studies involving a large number of animals. In contrast, noncannulation methods such as collection from the tail vein, orbital sinus, or jugular vein are most practical. Large volumes of blood can be obtained from the intact rat by cardiac puncture, although this method can cause shock to the animal system and subsequent death. Blood can also be obtained from sacrificed animals as described in the section on tissues and organs (p. 53).

Tail vein

Blood collection from the tail vein is a simple and rapid, nonsurgical method which does not require anesthesia. A relatively large number of serial samples can be obtained within a short period of time. However, this method is limited to relatively small sample volumes (≤250 μl per sample). Although larger volumes can be obtained by placing the rat in a warming chamber, this procedure could significantly influence the disposition of the test compound and therefore is not recommended for routine ADME studies. Despite the common concern of relatively low regional blood flow to the tail vein, blood collected from the cut tail has been shown to provide valid concentration data for numerous compounds.

The rat is placed in a suitable restrainer with the tail hanging freely. The tail is immersed in a beaker of warm water (37-40°C) for 1 to 2 min to increase the blood flow. Using surgical scissors or a scalpel, the tail is completely transected approximately 5 mm above the tip. The tail is then gently "milked" by sliding the fingers down the tail from its base. It should be noted that excessive "milking" could cause damage to the blood capillaries or increase the white cell count in the blood. A heparinized micropipet of desired capacity (25-250 μl) is held at a 30 to 45° downward angle in contact with the cut end of the tail (Fig. 3.6). This allows blood to fill the micropipet by capillary action. Application of gentle pressure with a gauze pad for ca. 15 sec is sufficient to stop bleeding. For subsequent sampling, the blood clot is removed with a scalpel. In this manner, a sufficient number of serial blood samples may be obtained to adequately describe the blood level profile of a compound.

If plasma is required, the blood may be centrifuged after sealing one end of the filled micropipet with a specially formulated vinyl plastic putty (Critoseal®) and placing it in a fiber glass padded centrifuge tube. The volume of plasma is determined by measuring the length of plasma as a fraction of the length of the micropipet, multiplied by the total capacity of the pipet. The tube is then broken at the plasma/red blood cell interface and the sample is expeled using a small bulb. If serum is needed, the blood should be collected without using anticoagulants in the sampling tube.

Orbital sinus

Serial blood samples can also be collected from the orbital sinus. In comparison with the tail-vein method, this technique permits rapid collection of larger (1-3 ml) samples. However, since it is recommended that light ether anesthesia be employed prior to each blood withdrawal, the method

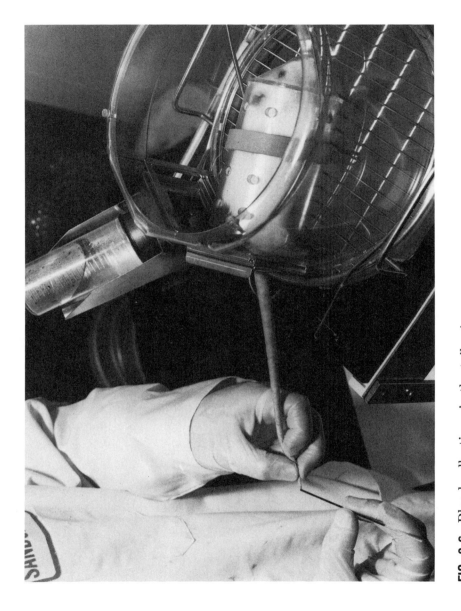

FIG. 3.6 Blood collection via the tail vein.

is cumbersome for most ADME studies in which frequent sampling is usually necessary.

The rat is anesthesized with ether until the corneal reflex is lost. Gentle pressure is applied to the eye causing the eyeball to slightly protrude (Fig. 3.7). A commercially available Pasteur pipet (approx. 14.5 cm) or microhematocrit tube for smaller samples is placed at the lower or inner corner of the eye and gently slid along the eyeball into the ophthalmic venous plexus which lines the back of the orbit (Fig. 3.8). The capillaries in this area are extremely fragile and thus they rupture upon contact with the tip of the pipet, filling the orbital cavity with a reservoir of blood. The accumulated blood immediately is drawn into the tube by capillary action. Once a pipet is in position, the actual bleeding time is about 1 to 2 sec. Bleeding usually stops immediately upon withdrawal of the pipet due to reestablishment of normal ocular pressure. Residual blood around the eye should be swabbed to avoid clot formation.

Although blood sampling from the orbital sinus often appears traumatic, this technique actually produces little or no animal stress even without the recommended anesthesia.

External jugular vein   A promising but less commonly employed method of obtaining serial blood samples from the intact rat is that of external jugular vein puncture as proposed by Gask and Barrett (4). This method requires no anesthesia, is rapid, allows for variable blood-volume collections, and is relatively stress-free.

The ventral neck and upper thorax are shaved. The animal is held securely in a supine position and

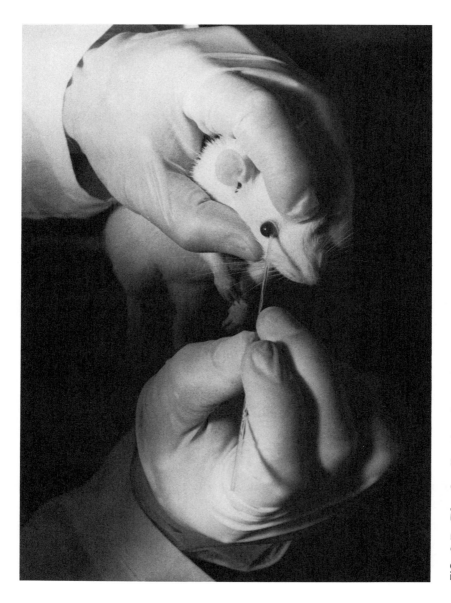

FIG. 3.7 Blood collection from the orbital sinus.

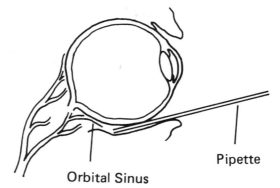

Pipette

Orbital Sinus

FIG. 3.8 Positioning of the pipette for blood collection from the orbital sinus. (Adapted from Ref. 3, with permission of *Proc. Soc. Exp. Biol. Med.*)

a 21 G needle attached to a syringe is inserted into the jugular vein (Fig. 3.9). When properly in place the needle will be oriented toward the top of the sternal bone with the syringe resting against the rat's jaw. Gentle withdrawal pressure is then applied to the syringe until sufficient blood has been obtained, after which the needle is carefully withdrawn. Alternate use of the left and right jugular vein allows serial collections of at least 6 samples per day.

Tissues and Organs

A major advantage of conducting ADME studies in rodents is the ease of obtaining concentration data in specific tissues and organs so that the overall distribution profile of the compound can be determined. This has particular advantage over studies in humans or larger animal species in which

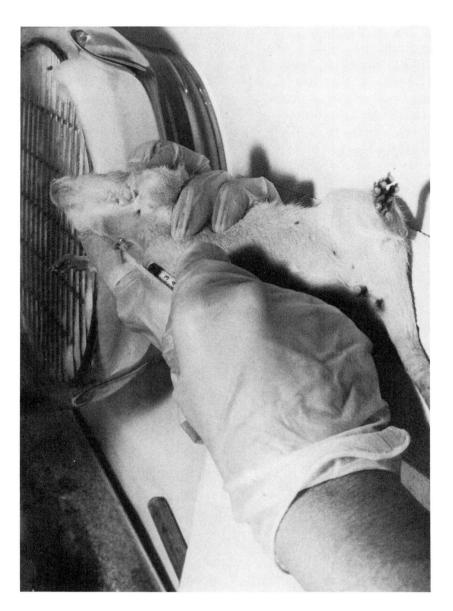

FIG. 3.9 Blood collection from the jugular vein.

sampling is usually restricted to the blood compartment. Due to analytical limitations such as the extraction of drug from small tissues and organs, however, only total radioactivity levels are examined in most distribution studies. Furthermore, since it is necessary to sacrifice the animal for tissue collection, serial sampling is not possible.

Standard distribution studies

Following ether anesthesia, the rat is placed on its back and a mid-line abdominal incision is made so that the inferior vena cava is exposed. A 22 G needle is inserted into the vein and as much blood as possible (approx. 10 ml for a 250 g rat) is withdrawn. The tissues and organs of interest should be carefully excised so that possible contamination from adjacent tissues is minimized. Samples that can be easily removed include the liver, lung, spleen, brain, kidney, heart, muscle, fat, testes, uterus, ovaries, adrenals, skin, bone marrow, lymph nodes, pancreas, salivary gland, thyroid, pituitary, eyes, epididymes, and the gastrointestinal segments, i.e., stomach and small and large intestines. The excised sample is rinsed with distilled water and blotted dry. Large organs, e.g., liver, kidney, spleen, etc., are homogenized (Polytron® , Brinkman) and aliquots used for analysis whereas smaller organs, e.g., adrenals and pituitary must be analyzed in their entirety.

Distribution in pregnant animals

Placental transfer studies are designed to examine the overall extent of fetal exposure to drugs that are administered to the pregnant animal. Since rats have a relatively short gestation period (22 days), these studies can readily be conducted during repeated drug administration throughout pregnancy so that any changes in distribution characteristics during the course of pregnancy can be examined. The ratio of the steady-state drug concentration in the fetus to that in the mother during chronic dosing is an index of relative drug exposure.

One male and one female rat of the same source and strain are mated in a cage. Mating is confirmed by the presence of vaginal plug, an approximately 3×5 mm coagulated mass of sperm, on the bottom of the cage or in the vagina. A vaginal smear is obtained and examined microscopically for spermatozoa only if no plug is found. The day of mating is generally considered day 0 of gestation. However, the finding of vaginal plugs or spermatozoa only indicates that mating has occurred and does not assure pregnancy.

The test compound is usually administered beginning on day 6 postconception (PC) and continuing through day 15 PC, which is an accepted period of dosing to cover organogenesis. Dosing prior to day 6 PC could kill the embryo before it implants.

Groups of animals are sacrificed during various stages of pregnancy, for example, at the same time after dosing on days 10 and 13 PC and after the final dose. Additional animals are sacrificed at designated times after the last dose in order to obtain an indication of the rate of drug removal from the body. A useful dosing and sampling schedule is shown in Table 3.1. Extra animals are mated and carried through the study to ensure the availability of a sufficient number of pregnant rats. This also allows for misdoses or spontaneous abortions.

At the designated sacrifice time, the rat is anesthetized and a ventral incision is made to expose the intestines, vena cava, and uterus. If the animal

TABLE 3.1 Design of a Placental Transfer Study in the Rat

Rats[a]	Days postconception											
	6	7	8	9	10	11	12	13	14	15	16	17
* * *	D[b]	D	D	D	DS[c]							
* * *		D	D	D	D	D	D	DS				
* * *		D	D	D	D	D	D	D	D	DS		
* * *		D	D	D	D	D	D	D	D	D	S	
* * *		D	D	D	D	D	D	D	D	D		S
* * * * *	D	D	D	D	D	D	D	D	D	D		
(extras)												

[a]Each * represents 1 rat.
[b]D = dose
[c]S = sacrifice.

is pregnant, blood is removed from the vena cava. The uterus is located and the fetuses in each horn that are not dead or resorbed are collected. A fetus is considered resorbed when decay and resorption into the mother's body is so extensive that anatomical features are no longer recognizable. The uterus with the ovaries attached is removed and placed on a wet paper towel on a watch glass. The ovaries are then separated. Next, the uterus is stretched across the watch glass and opened without damaging the amniotic sacs. The amniotic fluid is collected using a 1 ml syringe. Additionally, excretory organs such as the liver and kidneys are also obtained from the mother. The fetus is separated from the placenta, and the amniotic sac must be dissected from both. Finally, all extraneous tissues are removed from the uterus and discarded. Large organs are homogenized and aliquots used for analysis while smaller organs, e.g., ovaries, are analyzed in their entirety.

Excreta

Excretion samples commonly collected from the rat include urine, feces, bile, and expired air. By using properly designed cages and techniques, the samples can be completely collected so that the recovery of the administered dose (mass balance) is readily determined. These samples also serve to elucidate the biotransformation characteristics of the compound.

Urine and feces

These samples can be easily collected through the use of suitable metabolism cages. Since rodents are coprophagic, the cage must be designed to prevent the animal from ingesting the feces as it is passed. Other main features of the cage should include the ability to effectively separate urine from feces with minimal cross-contamination, a feed and water system that prevents spillage and subsequent contamination of collected samples, and collection containers that can be easily removed without disturbing the animal. Also, the cage should be designed so that it can be easily disassembled for cleaning or autoclaving. A commercially available product that appears to meet the above criteria is the Nalgene® Metabolic Cage (Fig. 3.10) although similar cages are also available from other manufacturers.

Following dose administration, rats are placed in individual cages. The urine and feces that collect in containers are removed at predetermined intervals. The volume of urine and the weight of feces are measured. After the final collection, the cage is rinsed, normally with ethanol or water, to assure complete recovery of excreta. If the rats are also used for serial blood sampling, it is important that bleeding be performed inside the cage to avoid possible loss of urine or feces.

Bile

The bile is the pathway through which an absorbed compound is excreted in the feces. In order to collect this sample, surgical manipulation of the animal is necessary. The anesthesized rat is placed on its back with its tail toward the investigator. Anesthesia is maintained throughout the surgical procedure. After shaving, a 1 inch midline abdominal incision is made posterior to the xiphoid cartilage. The duodenum with the bile duct is exteriorized through the incision. Two loosely tied loops are placed at each end of the bile duct approximately 0.5-1 cm near the hilum of the liver. A large bore needle threaded with PE-10 tubing (approx. 2 feet) is inserted through the back of the rat from inside the body cavity to the outside. The needle is subsequently removed. A small incision is made in the bile duct (Fig. 3.11) and the cannula is inserted. Beveling the end of the cannula facilitates insertion. Once the bile is flowing through the cannula, the duct is ligated using the two previously positioned loops, thereby holding the cannula securely in place. The intestinal loop is returned into the abdominal cavity and on top of the catheter, making sure bile flow is not obstructed. The abdominal muscle as well as the skin are closed with sutures. The rat is allowed to recover from anesthesia and then placed in a suitable metabolism cage. In order to minimize any potential effect of surgical trauma, a recovery period of at least 24 hours should be allowed prior to administering the test drug.

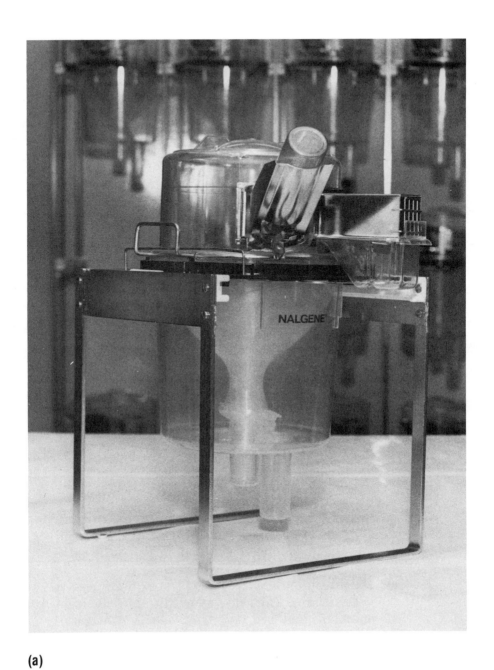

(a)

FIG. 3.10 Rat metabolism cages: (a) single- and (b) multiple-unit assembly.

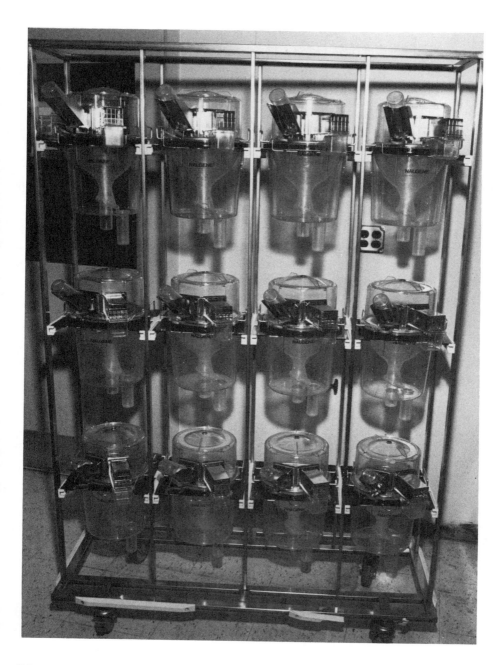

(b)

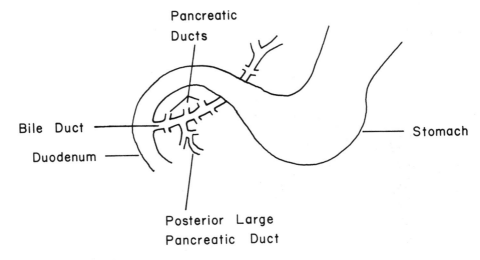

FIG. 3.11 Location of rat bile duct. (Adapted from Ref. 5, with permission of Academic Press.)

The cover of a standard metabolism cage unit (Maryland Plastics, Federalsburg, Maryland) can be modified to allow passage of the cannula while also serving as a restraint for the rat (Fig. 3.12). A clear plexiglas slab, 1.25 cm thick, is milled to fit the cage. Holes 1.0 cm in diameter are bored in the outer rim to allow air circulation. In a central opening an adjusting sleeve is positioned through which a piece of stainless steel tubing, 9.5 cm long, with an inner diameter of 6 mm and an outer diameter of 7.6 mm, is inserted. The portion of the tubing above the cover (6.5 cm) is fitted with an adjusting collar on a spring, which allows some flexibility in the length of the restraint for adaption to the rat's size and movement. A stop pin attached to the cover prevents tangling of the cannula while allowing 360° movement of the rat. The lower end of the stainless steel tube is inserted

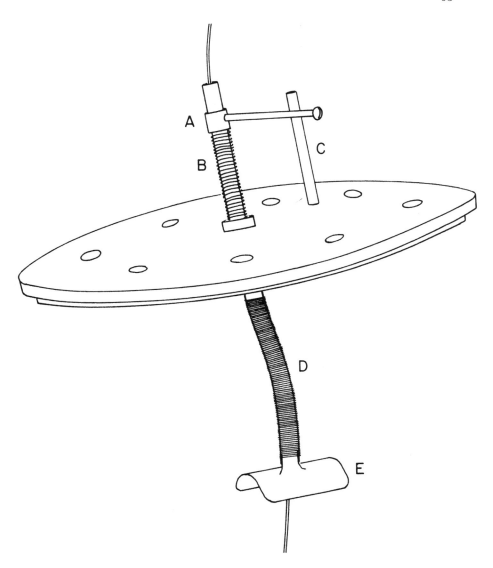

FIG. 3.12 Modified metabolism cage cover: A = adjusting collar; B = spring; C = stop pin; D = plastic hose protected by spring coil; and E = adaptor plate. (From Ref. 6, with permission of *J. Pharmacol. Methods.*)

into a flexible plastic hose (ca. 8 cm) that is fitted on a stainless steel adaptor plate (3.3 cm × 4.0 cm), curved to fit the contour of a rat's back. The plastic hose is protected by a spring coil. The bile duct cannula is passed through the stainless steel tube on the cage cover. The rat is then secured with adhesive tape to the curved adaptor plate, which should be centered over the incision where the cannula exits the rat's body. The free end of the cannula is connected to a suitable collection device. The cage modifications described above allow the rat freedom of movement for access to food and water. Additionally, urine and feces can be collected simultaneously.

A drug that is excreted in the bile enters the intestine, where some or all of the excreted dose may be reabsorbed to complete an enterohepatic cycle. Biliary secretion and intestinal reabsorption may continue until the drug is ultimately eliminated from the body via renal or fecal excretion or any other routes of disposition. A direct approach to quantitatively examine the effect of enterohepatic circulation on drug disposition is to monitor the biliary excretion and intestinal reabsorption in a "cascade" fashion. Thus, following drug administration, the bile obtained from a donor (dosed) animal is administered intraduodenally to a recipient animal, also with a bile fistula, and the excreta from both animals are collected and assayed. The bile ducts of a pair of rats (donor and recipient) are cannulated as described previously. Additionally, in the recipient rat, Silastic® tubing, 0.019 cm i.d., is inserted into the duodenum opposite the sphincter of Oddi and secured by ligation with surgical suture. The free end of the tubing is exteriorized through the incision at the back of the rat and passed through the cage cover assembly in the same manner as the bile duct cannula (Fig. 3.13). The bile from the

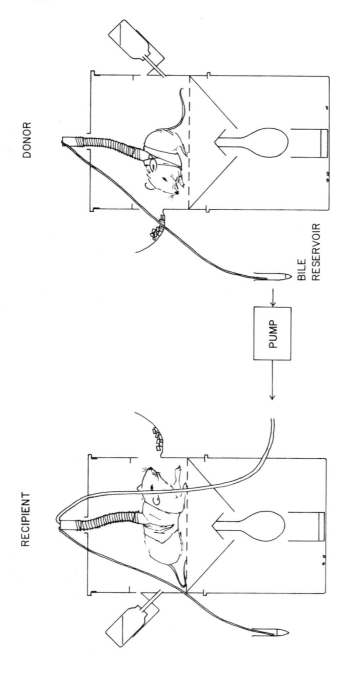

FIG. 3.13 Biliary excretion and intestinal reabsorption study. (From Ref. 6, with permission of *J. Pharmacol. Methods.*)

donor rat is collected in a 10-ml graduated centrifuge tube. After a reservoir of 1 ml has accumulated, the bile is delivered using a peristaltic pump
through a 0.013 cm i.d. Silastic® SMA tube into
the duodenal cannula of the recipient rat, at a rate
of 0.9 ml/hr. Since 250 g rats have a bile flow of
ca. 1 ml/hr, this reservoir volume will remain reasonably constant. Bile from the recipient rat as
well as urine and feces from both animals can be
collected at designated intervals for at least 3 days.

Expired air   For ^{14}C-labeled drugs, the tracer carbon may be
incorporated in vivo into carbon dioxide, a possi-
ble metabolic product. Therefore, when the position of the radiolabel indicates the potential for
biological instability, a pilot study to collect expired air and monitor its radioactivity content
should be conducted prior to initiating a full-scale
ADME study. Expired air studies should also be
performed in situations where the radiolabel has
been postulated to be stable but analyses of urine
and feces from the ADME study fail to yield complete recovery (mass balance) of the dose.

Following drug administration, the rat is placed
in a special metabolism cage (Fig. 3.14). Using a
vacuum pump, a constant flow of room air (approx. 500 ml/min) is drawn through a drying column containing anhydrous calcium sulfate (Dri-
erite®) impregnated with a moisture indicator
(cobalt chloride), and passed into a second column containing Ascarite® II, where it is ren-
dered carbon dioxide free. The air is then drawn
in through the top of the metabolism cage. Exhaled breath exiting the metabolism cage is passed
through a carbon dioxide absorption tower, where
the expired ^{14}CO$_2$ is trapped in a solution such as a

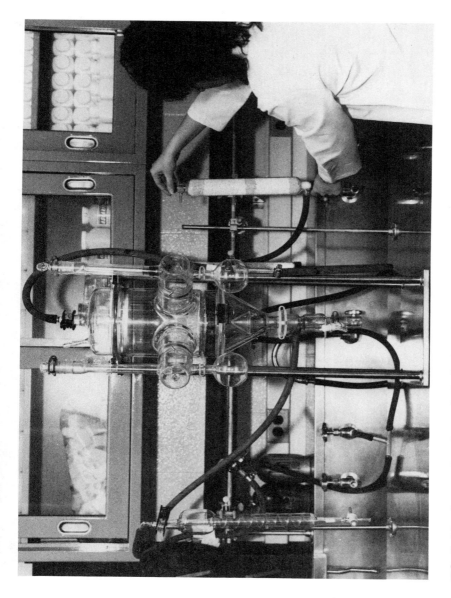

FIG. 3.14 Apparatus for exhaled air collection.

mixture of 2-ethoxyethanol and 2-aminoethanol (2:1). The trapping solution is collected, replaced with fresh solution, and assayed at designated times postdose so that the total amount of radioactivity expired as labeled carbon dioxide can be determined. The design of the cage shown in Fig. 3.14 also allows periodic collection of urine and feces without removing the rat from the cage.

Milk   The study of drug passage into milk serves to assess the potential risk to breast-fed infants in the absence of human data. The passage of drug into milk can be estimated as the milk-plasma ratio of drug concentrations at each sampling time or that of the AUC values. Approximately 30 rats in their first lactation are used. The litter size is adjusted to about 10 within 1 to 2 days following parturition. The test compound is administered to the mothers 8 to 10 days after parturition. The rats are then divided into groups for milk and blood collection at designated times postdose. All sucklings are removed from the mother rats several hours before milking. Oxytocin, 1 IU per rat, is given intramuscularly 10 to 15 min before each collection of milk to stimulate milk ejection. The usual yield of milk is about 1 ml from each rat. Blood is obtained immediately after milking. In order to minimize the number of animals used, the sucklings can be returned to the mother rat which can then be milked again 8 to 12 hours later.

References   1. H. B. Waynforth and R. Parkin, Sublingual vein injection in rodents, *Lab. Anim., 3*:35-37, 1969.

2. R. Sable-Amplis and D. Abadie, Permanent cannulation of the hepatic portal vein in rats, *J. Appl. Physiol., 38*:358-359, 1975.

3. V. Riley, Adaptation of orbital bleeding technique to rapid serial blood studies, *Proc. Soc. Exp. Biol. Med., 104*:751-754, 1960.

4. D. R. Gask and R. J. Barrett, Venepuncture-associated stress in the rat, Society of Toxicology 27th Annual Meeting, Dallas, Texas, February 15-19, 1988.

5. H. B. Waynforth, Experimental and Surgical Technique in the Rat, Academic Press, London, 1980, p. 128.

6. F. L. S. Tse, F. Ballard, and J. M. Jaffe, A practical method for monitoring drug excretion and enterohepatic circulation in the rat, *J. Pharmacol. Methods, 7*:139-144, 1982.

4

The Mouse

The mouse and the rat share many similarities with respect to their use in drug disposition studies. As described previously for the rat, mice can be easily obtained, housed, and handled. In fact, most experiments that are performed in the rat are carried out in a similar manner in the mouse. However, due to the relatively small size of the latter, serial blood sampling and surgical procedures such as bile duct cannulation are normally not attempted in the mouse.

Dosing

Oral

As is the case for the rat, oral doses in the mouse are usually given as a liquid (solution or suspension) or a drug-diet mixture. Liquids are administered using a small feeding needle (18 G, 1.5 in). With the thumb and index finger, the mouse is firmly held by the skin of its neck and back. The tail is held against the palm using the ring finger. The needle is gently inserted into the throat of the mouse so that the hub of the needle almost touches the mouse's teeth. The drug is then rapidly discharged. Severe struggling or appearance of the dose preparation in the mouth or nose indicates that the animal has been misdosed.

Drug-diet mixtures for mouse studies are prepared in an identical fashion to those used in studies in the rat. The specific drug-diet ratios, however, should be determined based on the average daily food consumption of a mouse, which is considerably less than that of the rat (approx. 6 g). Difference also exist between rat and mouse studies in the design of the cages due primarily to the difference in body size of these species. Specific mouse metabolism cages are commercially available although the Nalgene® Metabolic Cage for rats, shown in Fig. 3.10, can also be adapted for drug-diet studies in mice using a conversion kit which provides a smaller food hopper in addition to a smaller collection vessel and a support plate with a smaller grid. Similar cage modifications are also available from other manufacturers.

Parenteral   The most commonly employed parenteral mode of administration in disposition studies in the mouse is via the intravenous route. In order to select an appropriate site of injection, it should be noted that serial blood collection is usually not attempted in the mouse due to its relatively small body size and total blood volume. Instead, several mice are sacrificed at predetermined time points to generate statistically adequate data for depicting the concentration-time profile as discussed further in the following section. Consequently, a large number of animals need to be dosed in a single experiment. This normally precludes dosing through the jugular vein which needs to be surgically exposed for this purpose. On the other hand, since the mice are sacrificed for each bleeding, the tail vein is not required for blood sampling and thus becomes a suitable site for drug administration. The detailed procedure of dosing via the tail vein is virtually identical to that described previously for the rat.

Dosing via the portal vein is usually not attempted due to the difficulties associated with performing surgery on such a small animal. Other parenteral dosage routes, i.e., intramuscular, subcutaneous, can be used and these doses again are administered in the same manner as that described for the rat.

Biological Sample Collection

As discussed previously, serial blood sampling is usually not attempted in the mouse due to its small size. Thus, three or more mice are sacrificed at selected times for determination of blood concentrations. Tissue and organ collection is identical to that described for the rat, with the exception that the mouse possesses a gall bladder. Using appropriate metabolism cages, excreta also can be collected in the same manner as that discussed for the rat. However, bile duct cannulation is not attempted in the mouse.

5

The Dog

The dog is also a commonly used animal in drug metabolism and disposition studies since most research facilities are equipped to maintain and handle this species. Upon reaching maturity (7-9 months), the body weight of the dog is sufficiently stable over time to allow repeated studies in the same animal, i.e., studies using a crossover design. A distinct advantage of the dog over smaller species is the larger serial blood volumes that can be obtained. Approximately 100 ml of blood can be drawn from a 10 kg beagle every week for 6 weeks without significantly affecting its normal physiology. Another advantage of the dog is that oral dosage forms (e.g., capsules, tablets) intended for humans can generally be administered intact to dogs whereas this is virtually impossible in rodents. The large body size of the dog, however, also presents certain disadvantages such as the need for larger housing facilities and cages, greater amounts of test compounds, and somewhat greater difficulties in handling the animal. Additionally, inter-animal variability appears to be greater in the dog than in rodents. Due to ethical and economic considerations, tissue distribution studies are usually not conducted in this species.

Dosing

Oral

Either liquid or solid dosage forms can easily be administered to the dog. Liquids (solutions, suspensions) are prepared as previously described in Chapter 3. A practical dose volume in the dog is 1 ml per kilogram body weight. The liquid is given using a syringe and a flexible tubing, approx. 18" × 1/8" i.d. An 18 Fr. rubber urological catheter (Bard®) is suitable for this purpose. The dog's mouth is held open and the tube is carefully lowered into the stomach (Fig. 5.1). If desired, proper positioning of the tube in the stomach can be confirmed by placing the exteriorized end in a beaker of water. The appearance of air bubbles would indicate improper placement in the lung. Once properly positioned, the syringe filled with the liquid dose is attached and the dose injected into the stomach, usually over a 15 second interval. To assure complete delivery of the dose, the tubing should be flushed with water using the dosing syringe.

Solid doses are normally administered either as commercially available dosage forms (capsules, tablets, etc.) or as capsules filled extemporaneously with the test substance. For very small doses, it is convenient to incorporate a diluent such as lactose to aid in capsule preparation. This can be accomplished using a mortar and pestle, taking care to ensure uniform mixing. Empty gelatin capsules intented for humans can be used for relatively low doses while veterinary capsules (Michigan Capsule Company) are necessary for higher doses. For

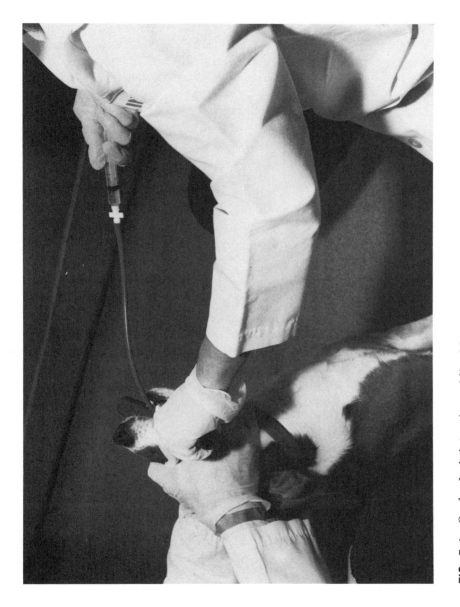

FIG. 5.1 Oral administration of liquids.

example, a No. 12 veterinary capsule can usually accomodate 1.5 to 2.0 g of loosely packed material. To administer the solid dosage form, the dog's mouth is held open and the tablet or capsule is placed on the posterior portion of the tongue so that it is not fractured or chewed before being swallowed. The mouth is then closed and the head tilted back for approximately one minute to assure swallowing. Gentle massage of the neck appears to facilitate this process. Normally the solid dosage form can be administered without water. In situations where fluid is desirable, such as to aid swallowing of large doses or dissolution of poorly soluble compounds, it can be given in the same manner as described previously for liquid dosage forms.

Emesis is a common problem in oral administration of drugs to the dog, which differs in this respect from the rat and the mouse. Due to the lack of an emetic center in the brain, rodents have no well-defined vomiting reflex. Thus in the dog, pilot studies should be conducted using a small number of animals (i.e., 1-2) to determine if the intended dose can be tolerated. If emesis occurs, parenteral antiemetics such as prochlorperazine or thiethylperazine can be administered although the potential of drug-drug interactions often renders this procedure undesirable. A better approach would be to lower the dose until the highest tolerable level is achieved. All pilot studies should be performed using nonradiolabeled drug to avoid the unnecessary use of radioactivity.

Parenteral

As discussed in the chapter on the rat, intravenous dosing is the most commonly employed parenteral route in ADME studies. The dose is normally prepared as a solution. As in the rodent, although pH, isotonicity, and sterility are factors that should be considered, they are not critical for a single administration if a small injection volume is employed. A typical volume for bolus injection in the dog is 0.1 to 0.3 ml/kg, while larger volumes would require slower infusion. The dose is normally delivered through a 21 G needle attached to a syringe. The use of a Butterfly® infusion set (Abbott) which consists of a 21 G needle connected to a flexible tubing often facilitates injection of the dose. Due to the relatively large size of the dog, a variety of veins including the cephalic (Fig. 5.2), femoral, jugular, and great saphenous veins can be used for dosing. These veins can be readily visualized by shaving the appropriate area. Injection is performed without surgical exposure so that anesthesia is not required under normal conditions. Following insertion of the needle, a small volume of blood is withdrawn to confirm that the needle is in the vein and the drug solution is then rapidly injected (approx. 15 sec). The needle is removed and gentle pressure is applied using a gauze pad at the injection site to minimize bleeding.

For the purpose of evaluating first-pass metabolism, the dose is administered via the portal vein. Under sterile conditions, the dog is anesthetized (e.g., intravenous xylazine, 2 mg/kg or ketamine, 5.5 mg/kg) and a midline abdominal incision is made. A silicon gum rubber tubing (Silastic®, Dow Corning), 0.076 cm i.d. and 0.165 cm o.d., is inserted into a tributary of the superior mesenteric vein near its junction with the portal vein, and is guided upward into the portal vein so that its tip projects several centimeters into this vein. It is then secured by ligation with suture. The part of the catheter inside the portal vein has a closed

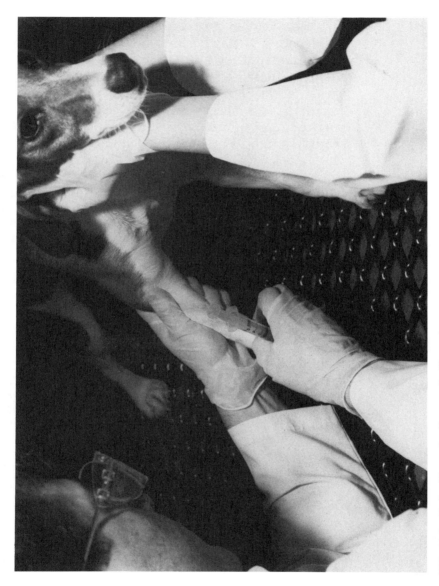

FIG. 5.2 Injection via the cephalic vein.

end with minute perforations so that intraportal doses can be delivered readily while clot formation is minimized without routine heparin injections. The other end of the catheter is passed subcutaneously and exteriorized through a stab incision at the nape of the neck, prior to closure of the abdomen with sutures. After recovery from surgery, the intraportal dose is administered by injecting directly into the catheter. If properly maintained, the catheter will remain patent for at least two months.

Another parenteral route of drug administration is by direct injection into an appropriate muscle such as the sartorius, gluteal, lumbar, and caudal thigh muscles. Intramuscular injection is relatively easy to administer and is generally less hazardous than intravenous doses since it does not result in a high initial blood level. The dose is usually administered using a 21 G needle inserted deeply into the muscle. The injection volume normally should not exceed 2 to 3 ml since larger volumes could result in pain and tissue damage as well as excessive leakage of the dose at the injection site. After dosing, the needle is withdrawn and a gauze pad is applied to the injection site to minimize drug loss.

Parenteral doses can also be administered by subcutaneous injection although this is not a commonly employed route. Using a 21 G needle, the vehicle is commonly injected into the area ventral to the thorax. Proper placement of the needle can be confirmed by feeling the tip through the skin. The dose is then delivered, the needle withdrawn, and a gauze pad applied to the injection site to reduce possible leakage.

Biological Sample Collection

Blood

In contrast to smaller species, relatively large blood samples can be frequently collected from the dog without altering its normal physiology. For example, 10 to 15 samples of 3 to 5 ml each can readily be obtained within the initial 24-hr period after dosing, followed by once or twice daily collections to adequately describe the blood level profile.

Serial blood samples can be obtained from the dog by direct venipuncture of the cephalic or femoral veins. Other veins such as the jugular veins can also be used. The blood is withdrawn through a 19 to 21 G needle attached to a Vacutainer® (Becton-Dickinson) or a syringe which has been flushed with heparin to prevent clotting. Although this is a relatively simple procedure, it is usually advisable to have a second person restraining the dog, especially if the animal has not been preconditioned. If urine and feces are being collected in the same experiment, blood sampling should be conducted without removing the dog from its cage.

Rapid blood collection at short intervals can be greatly facilitated by the use of an indwelling catheter. An infusion set (e.g., Butterfly®, Abbott) consisting of a 19 to 21 G needle connected to a flexible tubing is positioned in the vein. Clotting of blood in the cannula can be prevented by periodic infusion of 2 ml of saline containing approximately 20 U.S.P. units of heparin. Prior to each blood sampling, the residual fluid (blood, saline, and heparin) in the infusion set is withdrawn and retained. A new syringe is attached and blood is collected. The first syringe is then reattached and the residual fluid readministered.

Excreta

Urine and feces   Commercially available dog cages (e.g. Allentown Caging Equipment Co., Allentown, New Jersey) are usually suitable for the quantitative collection of urine and feces (Fig. 5.3). The gratelike design of the cage floor coupled with the tilted collection pan underneath permits reasonably good separation of urine and feces. The urine is drained through a tube into a collection vessel. If the test compound is known to be unstable in urine, the container can be placed in dry ice. Although this cage usually allows a quantitative estimation of urinary and fecal excretion, incomplete recovery of the dose could result if the dog urinates in the food or water pan or through the cage bars. Although these potential problems can be avoided by catheterization of the urinary bladder, this procedure requires special handling techniques and the use of anesthetics and could lead to infection.

Following collection and determination of the total volume, urine can normally be analyzed without further preparation. In contrast, fecal specimens must be further processed in order to yield a homogeneous mixture, in either dry or wet state. Feces can be dried in a conventional oven or a freeze-drier, the latter permitting the analysis of drug and/or metabolites that may be heat labile. Wet mixing is accomplished through the use of a specially designed laboratory blender. These techniques are described below:

1. *Oven-drying.* The feces is placed in an aluminum pan and dried in an oven until all moisture is removed. The material is then weighed and pulverized into a homogeneous mixture using a laboratory blender (e.g., Waring). Aliquots

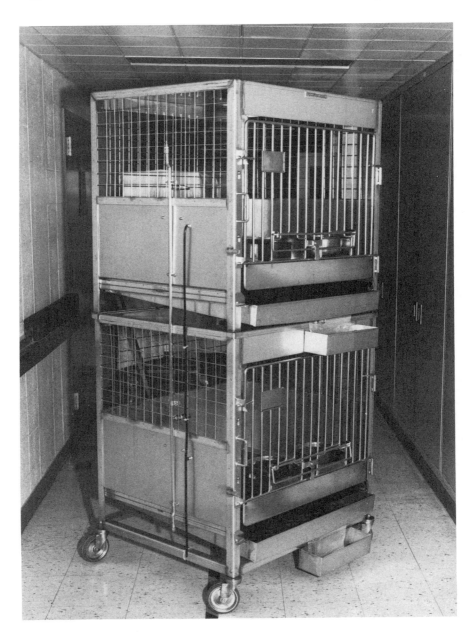

FIG. 5.3 Dog metabolism cage.

of the mixture are removed for analysis. Although oven-drying is a simple procedure, it requires special ventilation due to the nature of the sample. Additionally this technique is only suitable for determining total radioactivity since it is most likely that heat will affect the stability of drug and/or metabolites in the sample.

2. *Freeze-drying (lyophilization)*. Lyophilization overcomes the odor and stability problems often associated with using an oven, although the drying time is considerably longer (2-5 days). The feces is placed in the freeze-drier (e.g., Virtis, Gardiner, New York) in an aluminum pan. The material should be flattened to maximize the surface area in order to accelerate the drying process. The dried material is then weighed and pulverized into a homogeneous mixture for analysis.

3. *Wet-mixing*. The primary advantage of mixing fecal samples in the wet state is elimination of the lengthy drying process. Laboratory blenders specifically designed for the homogenization of feces are commercially available (Stomacher® Lab Blender, Seward Medical, London). The fecal sample is placed in a flexible (polyethylene) disposable bag and enough water is added so that a slurry will result. The total wet weight of the contents is determined. The container is then placed in the Stomacher, and the action of the machine transmits the necessary blending forces to the sample without coming into direct contact with it. Thus, no equipment cleaning is required. Mixing is usually complete within 2 min, and an aliquot is removed for analysis.

Bile

Bile is usually not collected in drug disposition studies in large laboratory animals such as the dog. In situations where direct biliary excretion data are required, several collection methods have been described. Using a special sampling technique, bile flow can be maintained for periods up to six months (1).

Reference   1. R. W. Marshall, O. M. Moreno, and D. A. Brodie, Chronic bile duct cannulation in the dog, *J. Appl. Physiol.*, *19*:1191-1192, 1964.

6

The Rabbit

The rabbit is the primary animal model used to investigate the teratogenic potential of new chemical entities. Thus, it is important to understand the disposition characteristics of the compound in this species. Of particular interest is the transfer of drug and metabolites across the placenta. Additionally, rabbits are commonly employed in the evaluation of topical dosage forms such as those intended for the skin and eyes.

As a laboratory animal for conducting ADME studies, the rabbit has certain distinct advantages in that it is relatively inexpensive and readily obtainable. Using proper restrainers, doses can be easily administered and blood samples collected. However, it should be noted that rabbits are more prone to contracting infectious diseases than other common laboratory species such as the rat and the dog. Also, the animal must be carefully handled to avoid fatal spinal injuries.

Dosing

Oral   For dose administration, the rabbit is placed in a
                  restraining device. For example, a Nalgene® rab-
                  bit restrainer (Fig. 6.1) is suitable for animals weigh-
                  ing from 3 to 4.5 kg, and is specially designed to
                  protect the rabbit from spinal injury. Animals
                  weighing more or less than the recommended
                  weights could sustain injury from struggling. The
                  chamber has a neck support which can be adjusted
                  in diameter and a butt plate which is adjustable
                  to vary chamber length. A stainless steel base in-
                  sert provides firm footing while allowing feces
                  and urine to drop into a removable base tray.

                  Either liquid or solid dosage forms can readily be
                  administered to the rabbit. Liquids (solutions,
                  suspensions) are prepared as previously described
                  in Chapter 3. A practical dose volume in the rab-
                  bit is 1 to 2 ml per kilogram body weight. The li-
                  quid is given using a syringe and a flexible tubing
                  approx. 16 × 1/8 inch i.d., such as an 18 Fr. rubber
                  urological catheter (Bard®). A plastic biting block
                  with a center opening is placed behind the upper
                  and lower teeth. The tubing is passed through
                  the opening and lowered into the stomach (Fig.
                  6.2). If the catheter is inadvertently inserted in
                  the lung, breathing through the tube will be audi-
                  ble. Another method of ensuring proper positioning
                  of the tube in the stomach is to place the end of
                  the catheter in a beaker of water; the appearance
                  of air bubbles indicates that the tube is in the lung.
                  Once the tube is properly positioned, the syringe
                  is attached and the dose administered. To assure
                  complete delivery of the dose, a small volume of
                  water is normally used to flush the tube.

                  To administer a tablet or capsule, the dosage form
                  is placed at one end of a flexible tubing, ca. 12 inches

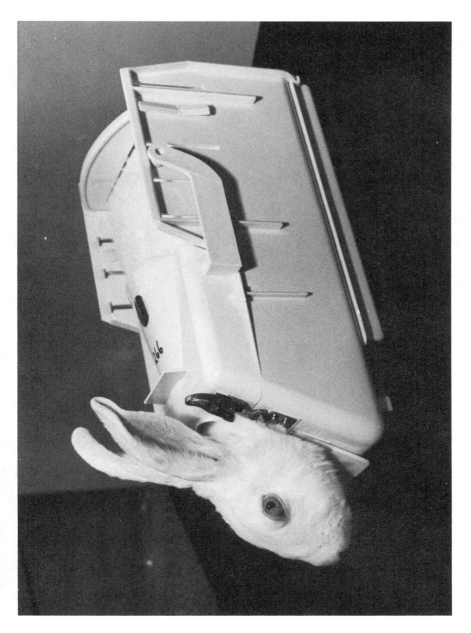

FIG. 6.1 Rabbit restrainer.

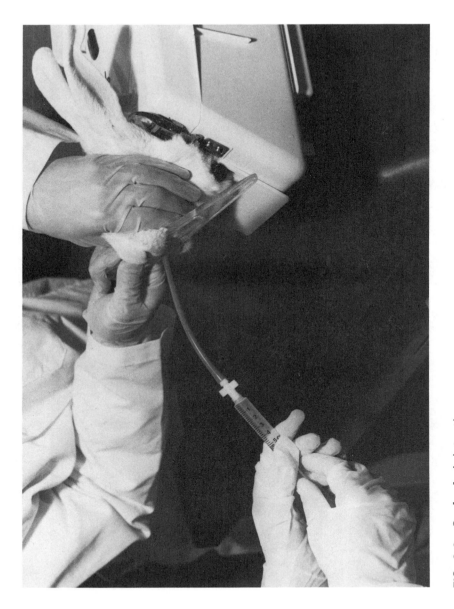

FIG. 6.2 Oral administration.

long. The urological catheter described previously
is suitable for this purpose after cutting off the tip
so that the tablet or capsule can be accommodated.
The dosage form should be fitted tightly enough
at the end of the tubing so that it remains in position during insertion into the stomach yet can still
be released from the syringe with a gentle stream
of air or water. To facilitate its ejection from the
tubing, the dosage form can be lubricated with a
small amount of vegetable oil.

Parenteral   Intravenous, subcutaneous, and intramuscular
administration are the most commonly employed
parenteral routes in the rabbit. Intravenous doses
are usually prepared in solution form. For acute
administration of relatively small volumes (approx.
0.3 ml/kg), the usual concerns pertaining to this
type of formulation (i.e., pH, isotonicity, sterility),
are not critical. The animal is placed in a rabbit
restrainer and the dose administered via the marginal ear vein (Fig. 6.3). If necessary, the ear can
first be shaved using a scalpel or electrical clipper
and the vein dilated by gentle rubbing. The dose is
normally delivered using a Butterfly® infusion
set (Abbott) which consists of a 21 G needle connected to a clear flexible tubing. The needle is inserted into the vein, bevel edge up. When the vein
is penetrated, a strong backflow of blood will appear in the flexible tubing. A syringe containing
the dose is then attached to the infusion set and
the drug injected. The plunger is drawn back slightly, and the appearance of blood indicates that the
needle was in the vein during the entire dosing
process. After removal of the needle, direct pressure is applied to the vein until bleeding ceases.

Subcutaneous doses are administered using a syringe and a 21 G needle. The skin on the rabbit's

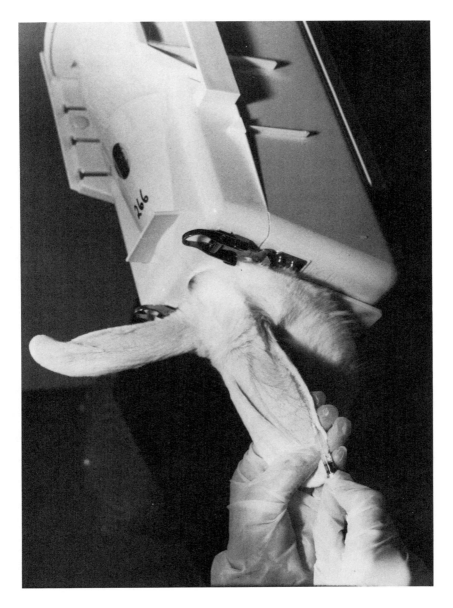

FIG. 6.3 Intravenous administration via the marginal ear vein.

back is lifted, and the dose is injected through the skin into the areolar connective tissue. The dose volume is similar to that used for the intravenous route, i.e., 0.3 to 0.4 ml/kg.

Intramuscular injections are usually given in the muscles of the hind-quarters, i.e. gastrocnemius or biceps femoris muscle. The hindlimb is shaved prior to injection. One technician securely holds the rabbit while another extends its hindlimb and administers the dose (Fig. 6.4). The appropriate dose volume, usually 0.25 ml/kg, is injected using a syringe attached to a 21 G needle.

Biological Sample Collection

Blood

Blood is usually collected from the veins of the ear. The rabbit is placed in a restrainer in which head movement is minimized. The marginal ear vein is dilated by gentle rubbing. A 22 to 23 G, 1 inch, heparinized needle is then inserted into the vein bevel edge up. Drops of blood will start to flow from the needle and can be collected directly into a heparinized tube or micropipette. To stop bleeding, the needle is withdrawn and gentle finger pressure is applied at the injection site. Approximately 10 serial blood samples of 1 ml each over a 24-hr period can be readily obtained using this method.

Since blood is likely to clot in the thin needle in the absence of an anticoagulant (e.g., heparin), the above method may not be suitable if serum samples are needed. Alternatively, a 5 mm incision can be made with a scalpel parallel to the marginal ear vein, and blood allowed to drip into an appropriate container. Collection is rapid,

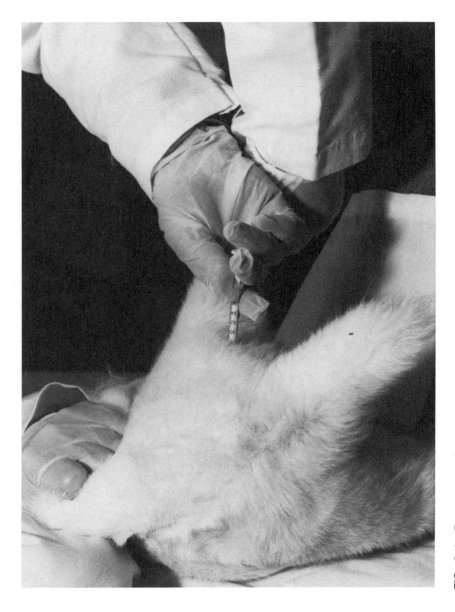

FIG. 6.4 Intramuscular injection.

usually 2 to 3 ml in less than 30 sec. Bleeding is stopped by applying a gauze pad and gentle pressure maintained by a clip. Prior to subsequent sampling, the wound is wiped clean with a wet gauze pad and bleeding starts spontaneously upon removal of the blood clot. This method is particularly useful for relatively frequent collections over a short period.

Tissues and Organs

Most tissue and organ distribution studies are performed in pregnant rabbits, primarily to assess the transfer of drug across the placenta. Since rabbits have a relatively short gestation period (31 days), these studies can be conducted during repeated drug administration throughout pregnancy so that any changes in drug distribution during the course of pregnancy can be examined. The ratio of the steady-state drug concentration in the fetus to that in the mother during chronic dosing is an index of relative drug exposure.

Table 6.1 describes a useful dosing and sampling schedule which covers the entire period of organogenesis and allows the evaluation of distribution characteristics at steady state. Extra animals are mated and carried through the study to ensure that a sufficient number of pregnant rabbits are available. This also allows for misdoses or spontaneous abortions.

Female rabbits are considered sexually mature when their vaginal area shows a dark purple color. For mating, a female is introduced into the cage of a male rabbit. To increase the likelihood of pregnancy, each female rabbit should be mated consecutively with two different males. The day of mating is generally considered day 0 of gestation. Since mating of all rabbits may not take place on the same day, the date of conception must be accurately recorded for each animal so that dosing and

TABLE 6.1 Design of a Placental Transfer Study in the Rabbit

Rabbits[a]	Days postconception														
	6	7	8	9	10	11	12	13	14	15	16	17	18	19	20
* * *		D[b]	D	D	DS[c]										
* * *		D	D	D	D	D	D	D	D	DS					
* * *		D	D	D	D	D	D	D	D	D	D	D	DS		
* * *		D	D	D	D	D	D	D	D	D	D	D	D	S	
* * *		D	D	D	D	D	D	D	D	D	D	D	D		S
* * * * * (extras)	D	D	D	D	D	D	D	D	D	D	D	D	D		

[a]Each * represents 1 rabbit.
[b]D = dose.
[c]S = sacrifice.

sacrificing will occur at the proper time. Alternatively, pregnant rabbits can be obtained from commercial suppliers.

As shown in Table 6.1, dosing usually begins on day 6 postconception (PC) and continues through day 18 (PC). Dosing prior to day 6 PC may kill the embryo before it implants.

At the designated sacrifice time, the rabbit is anesthetized by injecting sodium pentobarbital (0.5 ml/kg) into a marginal ear vein. The animal is then exsanguinated by cardiac puncture using a 20 G needle and a syringe. Subsequently, a ventral incision is made and the uterus located. The uterus with ovaries attached is removed and stretched across a 4 inch watch glass. The ovaries are then separated. Corpora lutea are dissected from the ovary and the number recorded. Each fetal pouch

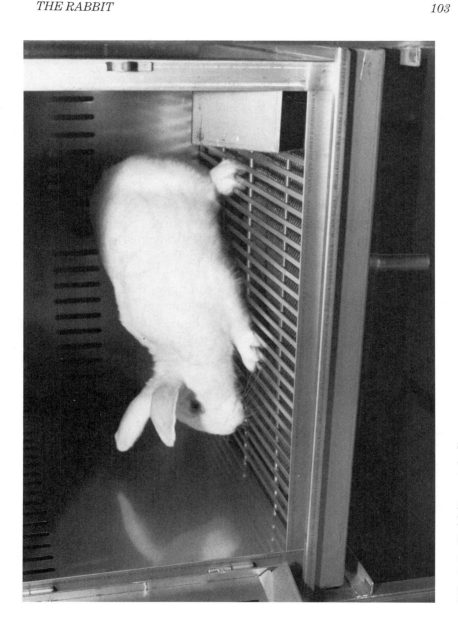

FIG. 6.5 Rabbit metabolism cage.

is opened. A 25 G needle attached to a 1 ml syringe is inserted into the amniotic sac and the amniotic fluid is gently aspirated from the inside sac. During the early stages of pregnancy when the amniotic sac is usually too small for aspiration, i.e., day 10 PC or before, the sac is cut and the fluid obtained from the watch glass. This method is less desirable than aspiration due to the greater possibility of contamination from other tissues. Next, the fetus is separated from the placenta, and the amniotic sac dissected from both. After all the fetuses, placentas, and extraneous tissues are removed, the uterus is rinsed with water and stored for analysis. Additionally, excretory organs such as the liver and kidneys are also obtained from the mother. Depending on the size of the different tissues at varying stages of gestation, they are analyzed either in their entirety or as an aliquot of the homogenate.

Excreta

Urine and feces can be quantitatively collected by housing the rabbit in a metabolism cage (e.g., Allentown Caging Equipment Co., Allentown, New Jersey, Fig. 6.5). Like rodents, rabbits are coprophagic and thus the animal must be prevented from ingesting its feces. Additionally, roughage should be incorporated into the animal's diet prior to and during the study to reduce the formation of trichobezoars (hairballs) in the gastrointestinal tract.

Following collection, the urine volume is measured and the sample is analyzed usually without further preparation. Fecal samples are normally homogenized in a laboratory blender (Stomacher® Lab Blender, Seward Medical, London) after the addition of a small amount of water, as previously described for the dog in Chapter 5.

7

The Monkey

The monkey is generally considered a good animal model for man in drug metabolism studies. Dosage forms intended for human use can readily be administered to the monkey. Due to its relatively large body size, the monkey can provide multiple serial blood samples over a short time interval.

It should be noted, however, that the use of monkeys in drug disposition studies is somewhat limited by the supply and cost of these animals. Monkeys also require special housing facilities and well-trained personnel for dosing and sample collection. Usually, at least two technicians are needed to control the animal during the experiment. Although the monkey can be sedated, e.g., using ketamine hydrochloride (Vetalar® , Parke-Davis, 5 mg/kg i.m.), this procedure is not recommended for drug disposition studies since potential drug-sedative interactions can occur. Furthermore, monkeys are a frequent source of serious human infection such as tuberculosis, rabies, B virus, salmonellosis, and shigellosis. Thus, those working with monkeys must have a thorough understanding of the potential hazards before any experiments are initiated.

Dosing

Oral

Prior to dosing, the monkey is removed from its cage and placed in a restraining chair (e.g. Plas Labs, Lansing, Michigan, see Fig. 7.1). The chair should be constructed in such a manner so that the restrained animal is in a comfortable position yet unable to harm the investigator. Additionally, the bottom of the chair should have a screened collection pan for the separation of excreta.

Oral doses (tablets, capsules, solution, suspension) are given using a syringe and a flexible tubing as described in Chapter 6 for the rabbit. A practical volume for liquid doses in the monkey is 1 to 2 ml per kilogram body weight. As in the rabbit, the tubing must be carefully positioned in the stomach in order to ensure complete and proper delivery of the dose (Fig. 7.2).

Parenteral

Intravenous doses are usually given to the monkey via the saphenous or femoral vein. The appropriate area is shaved while the monkey is seated in the restraining chair. The dose (approx. 0.1 to 0.2 ml/kg for bolus injections) is administered using a syringe attached to a 21 to 22 G needle. The needle is inserted into the vein bevel edge up. The plunger is withdrawn slightly, and the appearance of blood indicates that the vein has been successfully punctured. The dose is then rapidly injected. If relatively large dose volumes are necessary, they can be given by slow infusion. Following withdrawal of the needle, the injection site should be covered with gauze until bleeding ceases.

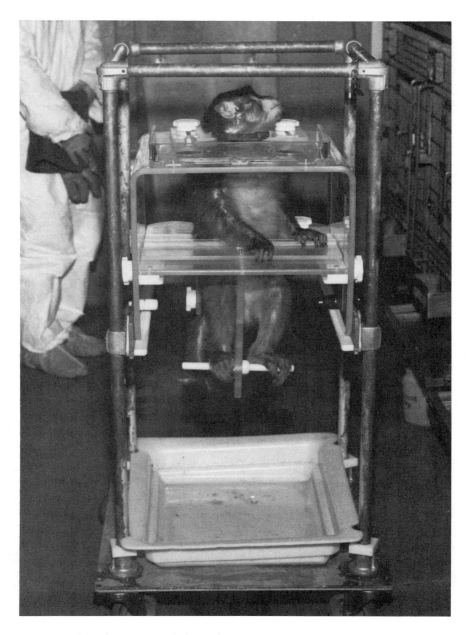

FIG. 7.1 Monkey restraining chair.

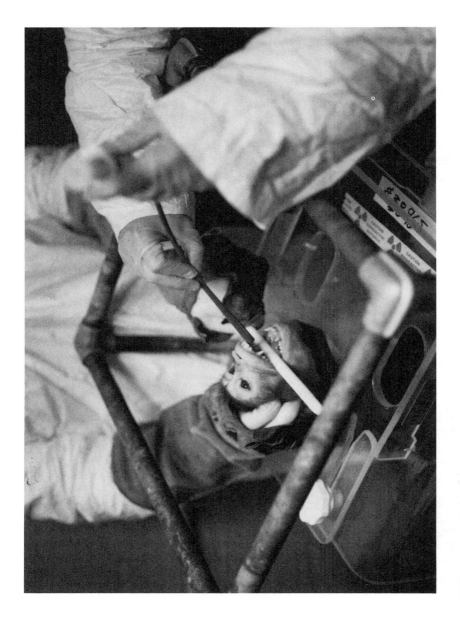

FIG. 7.2 Oral administration.

Subcutaneous doses can be given in the interscapular region while intramuscular doses are usually administered in the upper thigh muscles. The dose volume and needle size are usually the same as those utilized for intravenous administration in this species.

Biological Sample Collection

Blood   Due to the need for frequent blood sampling during the initial period after dosing (approx. 2 hr), the monkey is kept in the restraining chair. Blood can be collected from a number of blood vessels including the jugular, saphenous, and cephalic veins. A 21 G needle attached to a heparinized syringe is inserted into the vein, bevel edge up, and the blood is withdrawn. The sampling procedure may be facilitated by the use of a Butterfly® infusion set (Abbott). Following removal of the needle, a gauze pad is applied with gentle pressure until bleeding ceases.

When not seated in the restraining chair, monkeys are usually kept in specially designed "squeeze" cages (Fig. 7.3). A sliding partition is pulled forward and locked into position so that the animal is confined in the front end of the cage. The animal can be further restrained by using a pole with a hook at one end. After one technician has passed the hook through the monkey's neck collar, a second technician opens the front door slightly, firmly grasps a leg and extends it outside the cage. The leg is rotated until the saphenous or cephalic vein is visible. The blood is then collected as previously described. The front door of the cage is subsequently closed, the restraining hook released from the neck collar, and the sliding partition pushed back into its original positon, freeing the monkey.

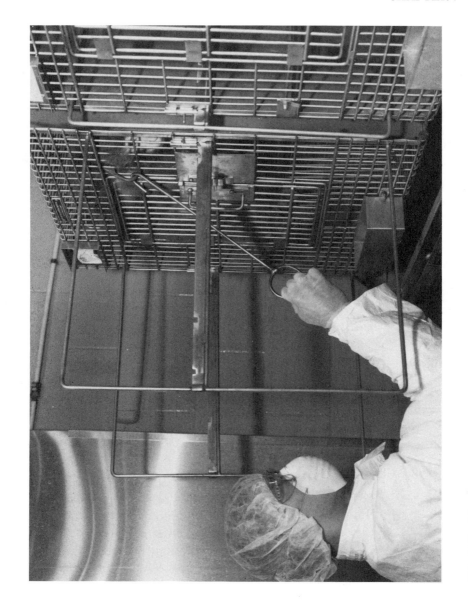

FIG. 7.3 Monkey squeeze cage.

Excreta

To collect urine and feces while the animal is seated in a restraining chair, the screened collection pan at the bottom of the chair is removed. The screen is detached and urine is poured into a suitable container. The feces are collected from the grid with tweezers. Since excretion may occur during this time, it is advisable to attach a second collection pan to the chair immediately after the first one has been detached for sample removal.

The "squeeze" cage is also suitable for the quantitative collection of excreta. The grate-like design of the cage floor coupled with the tilted collection tray underneath permits good separation of urine and feces. The urine is drained through a tube into a collection cup. The feces are removed from the tray with tweezers.

At the conclusion of the experiment, the restraining chair, the bottom and sides of the cage, as well as the collection tray are rinsed with water. Analysis of this cage wash is necessary to fully account for all drug-related material excreted by the animal. The urine and cage wash volumes are measured and the samples are analyzed normally without further preparation. Fecal samples are usually homogenized in a laboratory blender (e.g., Stomacher® Lab Blender, Seward Medical, London) after the addition of a small amount of water, as previously described for the dog in Chapter 5.

8

Data Interpretation

This chapter addresses the pharmacokinetic techniques that are commonly used to interpret the results of animal ADME studies. Since a limited number of animals (3-4 per experiment) are normally employed, the data should be viewed in a semiquantitative manner and caution must be exercised in extrapolating the findings to the species as a whole. For example, it might be more appropriate to describe the extent of drug absorption in a qualitative sense, i.e., poor ($<30\%$), moderate (30-60%), good (60-90%), or essentially complete ($>90\%$), rather than assigning a specific value, e.g., 78%. On the other hand, it should be recognized that despite the usually small 'N' (number of animals) in these studies, the reliability of the results are often comparable to human trials employing a greater number of subjects since experimental variables such as age, weight, strain, diet, housing, and sample collection can be more rigorously controlled in animals.

Absorption and Bio- availability

As previously defined in Chapter 1, absorption is the process by which a test compound and its metabolites are transferred from the site of absorption to the systemic circulation. In contrast, the term bioavailability concerns only the rate and extent to which the parent compound reaches the general circulation intact. Others such as the U.S. Food and Drug Administration have expanded this to include all active ingredients (active metabolites). In either case, bioavailability is distinctly different from absorption, which reflects the total exposure of the animal to the *parent drug as well as all drug-derived materials*. Thus, the measurement of total radioactivity can be used to assess drug absorption whereas a specific analytical method, e.g., HPLC, RIA, for the parent compound is only suitable for the determination of bioavailability. For an orally dosed compound, the difference between absorption and bioavailability could be due to chemical degradation in the gastrointestinal tract, microbial metabolism, gut wall metabolism, or presystemic metabolism in the liver.

The bioavailability of a compound can be estimated by comparing the blood or plasma level curves for the parent drug to those obtained from an intravenous reference dose. The rate of bioavailability is indicated by the time (t_{max}) required to achieve peak concentration (C_{max}), which can be obtained directly from the drug concentration-time curve. The extent of bioavailability is reflected by the area under the concentration-time curve (AUC), which is commonly calculated using the trapezoidal rule from time 0 to the last measurable concentration point. The residual area beyond this point can be estimated by assuming a log-linear decline as described in detail elsewhere (1). The ratio of the oral:intravenous AUC values is referred to as the absolute bioavailability of the compound and is normally used to characterize the disposition of the compound. Comparison of the AUC values of any two doses or dosage forms without an intravenous reference would indicate the relative bioavailability of these doses. The following example illustrates the determination of bioavailability for an experimental drug.

Example 1

In a typical ADME study of an experimental, cardiovascular drug in the rat, ^{14}C-labeled compound was administered orally at two dose levels and intravenously. Serial blood samples as well as cumulative urine and feces were collected and analyzed for total radioactivity and the parent drug. The blood level data are summarized in Table 8.1 and displayed graphically in Fig. 8.1. Relevant bioavailability parameters for the parent drug are extracted from the data and listed below:

Dose (mg/kg)	C_{max} (ng/ml)	t_{max} (hr)	AUC (ng·hr/ml)
8, i.v.	680	0.08	1700
8, p.o.	85.2	2	889
40, p.o.	640	4	5950

As expected, following intravenous dosing the maximum drug concentration was achieved immediately. The 8 and 40 mg/kg oral doses resulted in peak concentrations at 2 and 4 hour postdose, respectively, indicating a moderate rate of absorp-

TABLE 8.1 Blood Levels of Total Radioactivity and Parent Drug Following a Single Dose of a ^{14}C-Labeled Cardiovascular Agent

Time after dose (hr)	Radioactivity (ng equiv./ml)			Parent Drug (ng/ml)		
	8 mg/kg i.v.	8 mg/kg p.o.	40 mg/kg p.o.	8 mg/kg i.v.	8 mg/kg p.o.	40 mg/kg p.o.
0.083	700	–	–	680	–	–
0.5	520	31.2	118	402	14.5	42.3
1	317	68.2	370	220	31.6	130
2	250	165	850	167	85.2	325
4	185	220	927	96.5	77.9	640
6	114	170	982	72.2	64.3	520
8	93.0	142	800	56.0	49.8	364
12	78.5	94.5	550	35.1	28.4	192
24	58.2	56.7	281	8.08	5.24	29.7
32	43.7	46.2	198	*	*	9.24
48	30.0	28.4	132	*	*	*
56	25.1	23.3	108	*	*	*
72	16.6	14.1	70.3	*	*	*
96	8.82	7.90	37.4	*	*	*

*Below detection limit.

tion from both doses. The oral:intravenous AUC ratios, normalized by the respective doses, showed that the bioavailability of the parent compound was 52% after the 8 mg/kg oral dose and 70% after the 40 mg/kg oral dose. This difference could be due to dose-related alterations in either absorption or presystemic metabolism (first-pass effect). If only unchanged drug data are obtained, these potential causes cannot be differentiated.

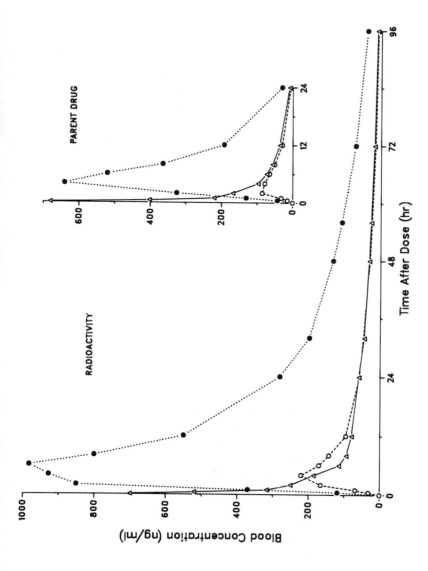

FIG. 8.1 Blood levels following a single dose (△, 8 mg/kg i.v.; ○, 8 mg/kg p.o.; ●, 40 mg/kg p.o.) of a ¹⁴C-labeled cardiovascular agent. The radioactivity concentrations are expressed in terms of ng equivalents of the parent drug per milliliter.

Dosing with radiolabeled compound enables the determination of total drug absorption in intact animals so that the processes of absorption and presystemic metabolism can be distinguished. Absorption is usually determined using all available sources of information including blood levels as well as urinary, biliary, and fecal excretion.

1. *Blood levels.* Using the concentration data for total radioactivity in Example 1 (Table 8.1), the absorption parameters are derived and listed below:

Dose (mg/kg)	C_{max} (ng equiv/ml)	t_{max} (hr)	AUC (ng equiv·hr/ml)
8, i.v.	700	0.08	5110
8, p.o.	220	4	4680
40, p.o.	982	6	23600

Similar to the unchanged drug data, the peak radioactivity concentration following the high dose was achieved at a later time than after the low dose. The extent of absorption, calculated from the oral:intravenous AUC ratio and normalized by the dose, was 92% for both oral doses.

In the above interpretation, it should be stressed that the blood levels of total radioactivity do not represent a single component but are a composite of the parent drug and all circulating metabolites. Thus, for the cardiovascular drug in this example, the concentration of total radioactivity equals the sum of the concentrations of unchanged drug and two metabolites, as illustrated in Fig. 8.2 using the low (8 mg/kg) dose data. In order to use the *concentration* (and thus, AUC) data of total radioactivity to estimate the *amount* of drug and/or metabolites absorbed, all the systemically circulating radiolabeled components (i.e., drug and metabolites) need to have identical apparent volumes of distribution. Under normal circumstances where this cannot be readily established, the radioactivity AUC ratio would be a valid absorption index only if the drug undergoes little or no first-pass metabolism and the doses studied do not saturate the usual elimination pathways. On the other hand, if the metabolite mix after intravenous dosing is substantially different from that following an oral dose, the oral:intravenous AUC ratio of total radioactivity can be smaller than, equal to, or even greater than unity, depending on the distribution characteristics of each radiolabeled component and regardless of the extent of absorption from the oral dose. Therefore, there is clearly some uncertainty in absorption estimates that are based solely on AUC ratios of blood radioactivity. For more accurate assessments of total drug absorption, the blood level data should be used in conjunction with other observations made in the same experiment.

2. *Urinary excretion.* The ratio of cumulative urinary recovery of radioactivity after oral and intravenous drug administration is a commonly accepted index of absorption. Thus, using the excretion data shown in Table 8.2, the absorption of the cardiovascular drug discussed in the Example above was 60.9/68.0 = 90% from the low oral dose and 62.8/68.0 = 92% from the high oral dose. Naturally, this method is only valid provided that the excretion pattern (urine: feces ratio) of *absorbed* radioactivity does not

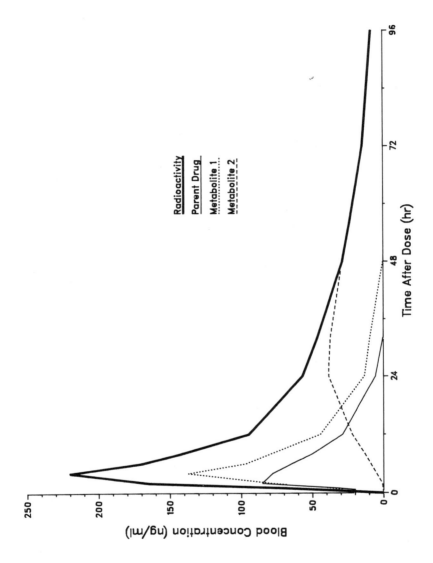

FIG. 8.2 Blood levels following a single oral dose (8 mg/kg) of a ^{14}C-labeled cardiovascular agent. Metabolite and radioactivity concentrations are expressed in
terms of ng equivalents of the parent drug per milliliter.

TABLE 8.2 Excretion of Total Radioactivity Following a Single Dose of a ^{14}C-Labeled Cardiovascular Agent

	Time interval (hr)	Percent of dose		
		8 mg/kg i.v.	8 mg/kg p.o.	40 mg/kg p.o.
Urine	0-24	62.8	56.0	60.5
	24-48	3.0	2.9	1.3
	48-72	1.4	1.4	0.7
	72-96	0.8	0.6	0.3
	0-96	68.0	60.9	62.8
Feces	0-24	11.7	28.7	11.9
	24-48	5.3	3.1	15.0
	48-72	2.0	0.9	2.4
	72-96	1.8	0.4	0.8
	0-96	20.8	33.1	30.1
Cage wash	0-96	2.0	0.6	0.5
Total	0-96	90.8	94.6	93.4

vary significantly with dose and route of administration. For example, if a substantial portion of the oral dose is absorbed in the form of a metabolite resulting in a urinary:fecal radioactivity ratio different from that following intravenous dosing, the oral:intravenous quotient cannot be used as a means of estimating absorption. Under all circumstances, however, the urinary recovery of an orally administered radioactive dose can still provide useful information as it represents the minimum amount of drug absorbed. Thus, in the present example (Table 8.2), it can be stated with confidence that a minimum of 61% and 63% of the low and high oral doses, respectively, were absorbed.

3. *Parent drug in feces.* Excluding biliary excretion of intact drug, any intact drug recovered in the feces can generally be assumed to represent the unabsorbed portion of the dose. For the cardiovascular drug discussed in Example 1, the parent compound was analyzed in cumulative urine and feces and the results given in Table 8.3. The data would suggest that 94% of the low oral dose and 92% of the high dose were absorbed. However, owing to the possibility of drug metabolism in the gut epithelium or by intestinal microflora, the actual amount unabsorbed could be considerably greater. Therefore, absorption estimates obtained from this method should be applied in a qualitative manner. The method should not be used as the sole index of absorption but may serve as a secondary, supportive indicator.

4. *Biliary excretion.* If properly conducted to maintain physiologic conditions, experiments using bile duct-cannulated animals can yield definitive information concerning the extent of drug absorption. Following oral administration of a radiolabeled compound, the total recovery of radioactivity in urine and bile would indicate the minimum amount of drug absorbed;

TABLE 8.3 Excretion of Parent Drug Following a Single Dose of a ^{14}C-Labeled Cardiovascular Agent

	Time interval (hr)	Percent of dose		
		8 mg/kg i.v.	8 mg/kg p.o.	40 mg/kg p.o.
Urine	0-96	19.9	15.2	18.6
Feces	0-96	0.2	5.6	8.1

any radioactive material present in feces would probably represent unabsorbed drug. For example, when administered orally (8 mg/kg) to rats with bile fistulae, the cardiovascular agent in Example 1 yielded the excretion profile shown in Table 8.4. By calculating the sum of biliary and urinary excretion, absorption was estimated to be minimally 80%. It should be noted, however, that this value often represents an underestimate of drug absorption due to the depletion of bile from the animal during the experimental process. Since bile salts are needed for the solubilization of numerous drugs in the gastrointestinal tract, they can play an important role in the absorption of these compounds.

TABLE 8.4 Excretion of Radioactivity Following a Single Oral Dose (8 mg/kg) of a ^{14}C-Labeled Cardiovascular Agent to Bile Duct-Cannulated Rats

	Time interval (hr)	Percent of dose
	0-2	3.5
	2-6	7.2
Bile	6-24	14.3
	24-48	2.2
	0-48	27.2
Urine	0-48	53.0
Feces	0-48	12.4
Cage wash	0-48	1.1
G.I. tract	48	1.8
Total	0-48	95.5

Usually a combination of two or more of the absorption indices described above will provide an accurate assessment of the extent of absorption. Based on the results obtained from these various approaches as summarized in Table 8.5, it can be concluded that the absorption of the cardiovascular drug studied is greater than 90% at both dose levels and is therefore considered to be virtually complete.

While blood concentration analysis can reveal the onset and rate of drug absorption, the oral:intravenous urine quotient in intact animals is a more reliable indicator of the extent of absorption, especailly for drugs that are predominantly excreted in urine. This method may not be appropriate if the renal route represents only a minor pathway of drug excretion, since any experimental error in urine collection or analysis would tend to result in relatively large deviations in absorption estimates. The bile duct-cannulated animal

TABLE 8.5 Absorption of a Cardiovascular Agent Estimated Using Different Parameters

		Percent of dose absorbed	
Parameter	Method of calculation	8 mg/kg	40 mg/kg
Blood	$AUC_{p.o.}/AUC_{i.v.}$	92	92
Urine	$Urine_{p.o.}/Urine_{i.v.}$	90	92
Feces	100% - % dose recovered unchanged in feces	94	92
Bile and urine	% dose recovered in bile + % dose recovered in urine	>80	—

model is also useful for the assessment of the extent of absorption. The disadvantages associated with this method, however, are the necessity of surgical intervention which could induce stress in the animal, and the depletion of bile during the experimental period. both of these factors could result in altered absorption or disposition patterns.

Distribution   The concentrations of drug-related material (total radioactivity) in major tissues and organs reveal the degree of transient exposure of specific organs to the drug. The distribution data for a CNS (central nervous system) drug in the rat are graphically presented in Fig. 8.3. To facilitate the comparison of results obtained following a low and a high oral dose, the tissue concentrations are dose-normalized. As one would expect in a typical distribution study, the highest concentrations of radioactivity were observed shortly after dosing in the well-perfused, excretory organs, i.e., the kidneys and liver. At the same sampling time, blood and other tissues showed lower, albeit substantial, levels. Overall there appeared to be no dose-related differences in the distribution of this compound. Twenty-four hours after oral administration, both the low and high oral doses showed tissue concentrations less than 5% of the respective early values, indicating little or no retention of drug-related material.

Another important role of distribution studies is to investigate the potential for drug accumulation in the tissues. From serially collected tissue samples following a single dose, an estimation of the overall rate of decline of radioactivity can be

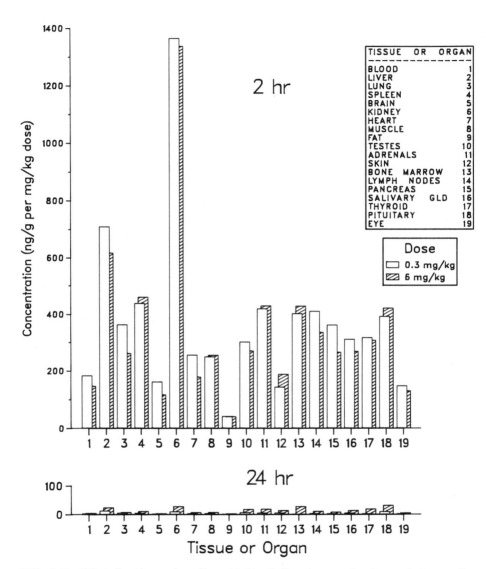

FIG. 8.3 Distribution of radioactivity following a single oral dose of a
[14]C-labeled CNS drug. Radioactivity concentrations are expressed in
terms of ng equivalents of the parent compound per gram, normalized
by the dose.

obtained using a semi-logarithmic plot as shown in Fig. 8.4 for the CNS drug. Each curve represents one of the tissues previously described in Fig. 8.3. In this example, the longest half-life was approximately 85 hours. Based on the following equation,

$$\text{Accumulation Ratio} = \frac{1}{1 - e^{-0.693\tau/t_{1/2}}} \qquad (8.1)$$

where τ is the dose interval and $t_{1/2}$ is the half-life, it can be estimated that the concentrations in the tissues following multiple daily administration would be no more than 5 to 6 times those obtained after a single dose. This can then be verified by a multiple dosing study in which the drug is repeatedly given until the concentrations reach a plateau, i.e., steady state. The time required to approach steady state during a multiple-dosing regimen is independent of the dose frequency, or input rate, and is dependent solely on the elimination half-life of the drug. Specifically, concentrations would be essentially at steady state after repeated dosing for approximately five half-lives (2) or, in this example, two weeks or less depending on the tissue. Normally the trough concentration, i.e., the concentration immediately prior to the next dose, at steady state ($C_{min(ss)}$) is compared to that following the initial dose ($C_{min(1)}$), as shown in Fig. 8.5. As expected, the trough concentration was higher following multiple dosing than after the first dose, the accumulation being 5 to 6 times in some tissues.

Metabolism   In addition to total radioactivity and parent drug data, information on the metabolism of the com-

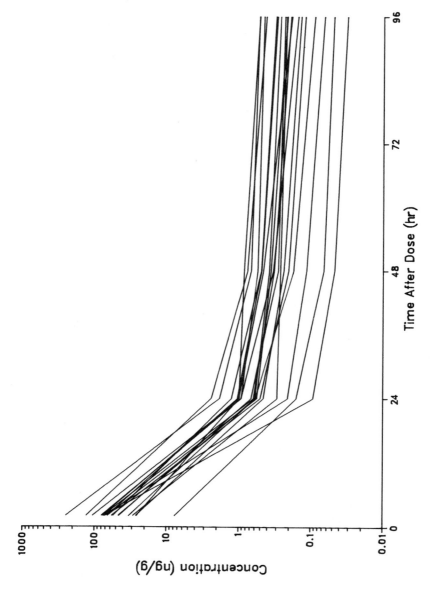

FIG. 8.4 Tissue concentrations of radioactivity, expressed in terms of ng equivalents of the parent drug per gram, following a single oral dose (0.3 mg/kg) of a ^{14}C-labeled CNS drug. Each curve represents one tissue.

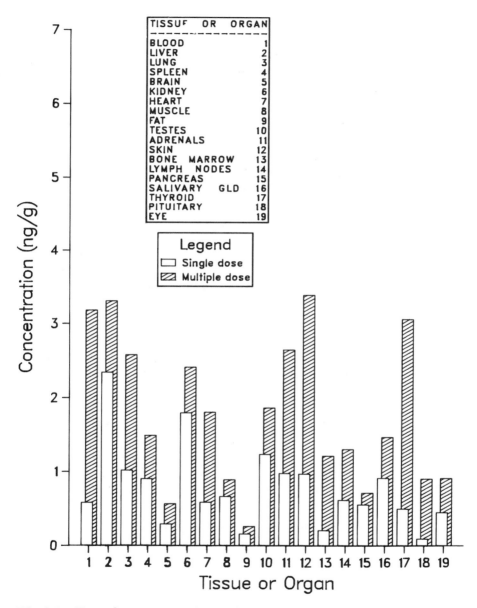

FIG. 8.5 Trough concentrations of tissue radioactivity, expressed in terms of ng equivalents of the parent drug per gram, after a single dose and during multiple dosing (0.3 mg/kg/day) of a ¹⁴C-labeled CNS drug.

pound is also obtained in a typical ADME study. Minimally these studies will yield metabolite patterns in biological samples, usually blood/plasma, urine, bile, and feces. Although a number of methods have been used for quantitative metabolic profiling, complete accounting of all constituents in the particular sample can be assured only by techniques which utilize radioactive specimens, i.e., those obtained following the administration of a radiolabeled drug. One such procedure is high pressure liquid chromatography with on-line radioactivity monitoring (HPLC/RAM) which allows for the separation and quantification of biotransformation products. The chromatographic peaks, measured in disintegrations per minute (dpm) and each representing a different metabolite, are usually assigned numbers in the order of their elution from the chromatographic column. The amount of radioactivity in each peak can be expressed as a percent of the total radioactivity in the specimen. The sum of all the peaks represents the fraction of total radioactivity that is quantifiable. The portion not quantifiable is probably due to incomplete extraction procedures and/or minor metabolite peaks below the limit of detection. An example is given in Fig. 8.6 which shows the urinary metabolite patterns for a cholesterol lowering agent in five species. A total of ten metabolites were characterized and numbered according to their retention times.

A primary objective of metabolism studies in animals is to identify those species which can serve as a model for man. In most cases, two or more species are necessary to encompass the complete spectrum of metabolites observed in man. In the above example (Fig. 8.6), parent drug and three quantifiable metabolites (peaks 4, 9, and 10) were

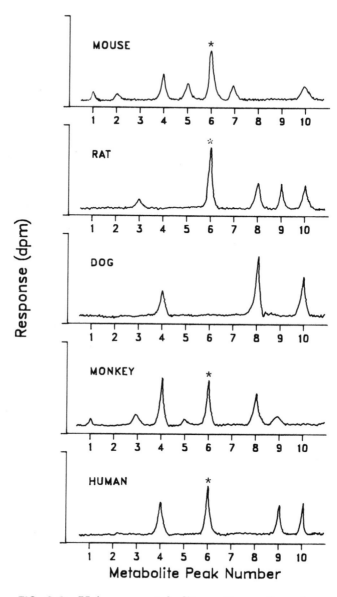

FIG. 8.6 Urinary metabolite patterns for a hypocholesterolemic agent in five species. Asterisk indicates the parent drug.

found in human urine. These four peaks were also seen in at least one animal species, although no single animal appeared to be an adequate model for man. Nevertheless, the mouse and rat together produced all the human metabolites and thus it would be logical to confine further metabolism work on this compound to these two species. Usually, additional studies are conducted to identify the major metabolite peaks, using such methods as nuclear magnetic resonance (NMR) and mass spectrometry (MS). The specific details of these techniques are beyond the scope of this text.

It should be noted that chronic administration of a drug can result in altered biotransformation due to enzyme induction or inhibition. Thus, metabolism studies should be performed under both acute and chronic dosing conditions.

Excretion

One of the primary objectives of ADME studies is to demonstrate that the administered dose is excreted from the body in a reasonable time period. By using radiolabeled drug, it is possible to determine if the dose is completely eliminated (i.e., achieving mass balance). Failure to recover a substantial portion ($>85\%$) of the administered radioactivity could indicate errors in dosing, collection, or analysis, tissue retention of radioactivity, or metabolic instability of the radiolabel. All of these possibilities should be considered to assure the validity of the results.

One unique route of drug excretion in lactating animals is via the breast milk. The use of animal models enables the prediction of drug exposure in breast-fed infants. First, the serial drug concentrations in milk and plasma of the animal model are used to calculate the respective AUC values, the ratio of which indicates the extent of drug passage into milk. This ratio is then applied to the average plasma concentration in humans to obtain the average milk level following a given dose. Based on an approximate milk consumption of 150 ml/kg per day by an average infant, the quantity of drug received via the milk can be readily calculated. For example, if data in the rat show a milk-plasma drug AUC ratio of 5, an average plasma concentration of 1 ng/ml observed in a nursing mother following a 5 mg dose would correspond to an average milk level of 5 ng/ml. Therefore, the maximum amount of drug that an infant could be exposed to by ingesting 1 liter of milk per day would be 5 μg, i.e., about 0.1% of the adult dose.

By quantitative collection of excreta at sufficient frequency, it is possible not only to provide information on the overall excretion pattern, that is, percentage of dose in urine, bile, and feces, but also to allow an assessment of the rate of elimination. Usually the elimination rate of a drug is evaluated in terms of its terminal half-life ($t_{1/2}$) in blood (or plasma/serum), which can be defined as the time required for the concentration of drug to be reduced by a factor of two. The half-life is particularly useful in estimating the time required to reach steady-state blood levels and also the degree of accumulation during a given dosing regimen. Although half-lives can be calculated by curve-fitting of data using sophisticated computer programs, a simple and rapid method of determining half-lives is by plotting the blood concentration versus time data on semilogarithmic paper to establish the terminal, log-linear phase of the curve.

A linear regression analysis of the data points constituting this phase is performed so that the line of best fit can be drawn. The half-life is subsequently determined directly from the line as shown in Fig. 8.7, or by using the following equation:

$$t_{1/2} = \frac{0.693}{-K} \tag{8.2}$$

where $-K$ is the slope of the straight line. Applying either procedure to the data for the cardiovascular drug in Example 1 (Table 8.1), the half-lives following the intravenous and low and high oral doses, respectively, are estimated to be 26, 25, and 25 hours for total radioactivity and 5.6, 5.0, and 4.5 hours for the parent drug. Thus, the time to reach steady-state blood radioactivity levels would be approximately 125 hours (i.e., five half-lives). The degree of accumulation can be calculated using the following equation:

$$\text{Accumulation ratio} = \frac{1}{1 - e^{-K\tau}} \tag{8.3}$$

where τ is the dose interval. For the cardiovascular drug in Example 1, the accumulation upon multiple dosing (8 mg/kg, p.o., once daily) would be approximately twofold, as shown in Fig. 8.8.

The key to success with the above method of half-life determination lies entirely in properly defining the terminal phase. As shown in Fig. 8.9, the true terminal phase is likely to be missed if blood samples are not collected for an adequate length of time or if a relatively insensitive assay procedure is used. These circumstances usually result in an underestimate of the elimination half-life. On the other hand, due to the recent development of sensitive analytical methods, e.g., GC-MS, RIA, re-

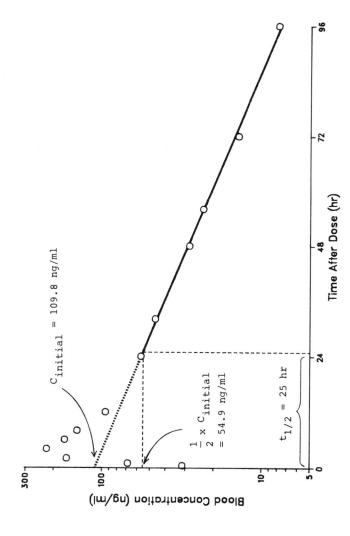

FIG. 8.7 Half-life determination. The blood levels represent total radioactivity, expressed in ng equivalents of the parent drug per milliliter, following an oral dose (8 mg/kg) of a ^{14}C-labeled cardiovascular drug (see Table 8.1).

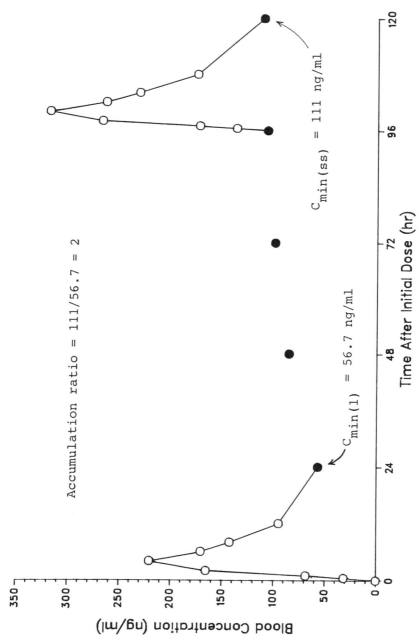

FIG. 8.8 Blood levels of radioactivity, expressed in ng equivalents of the parent drug per milliliter, during multiple daily administration (8 mg/kg/day, p.o.) of a ^{14}C-labeled cardiovascular drug. Closed circles represent blood levels immediately preceding each successive dose, i.e., $C_{min(1)}, \cdots C_{min(ss)}$.

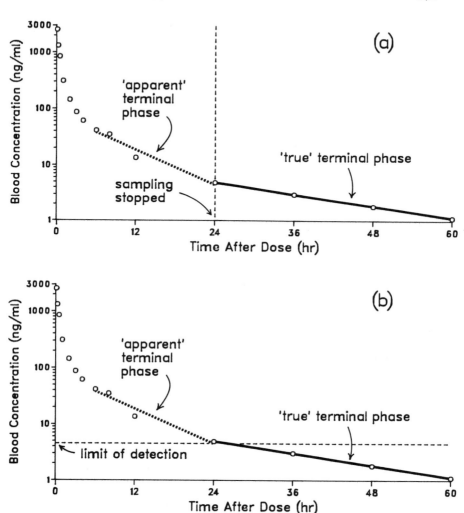

FIG. 8.9 The true terminal phase (half-life = 17 hr) would be missed if (a) blood samples are not collected for an adequate length of time or, (b) if the assay method lacks sensitivity. Either circumstance would result in an apparent terminal half-life of 5.8 hr, a considerable underestimate.

liable measurements can be obtained even at very low concentrations. This often results in a terminal phase of low but lasting blood levels and, therefore, a relatively long half-life. The significance of the terminal half-life, however, must be interpreted in terms of its potential contribution to drug accumulation. A simple method used to evaluate the relevance of a particular half-life is to calculate its contribution to the total AUC (3). The blood levels of most drugs can be described by a polyexponential equation. For example, if three exponential terms are required to describe the data, the following equation represents the time course of the blood concentration, C:

$$C = A_1 e^{-K_1 t} + A_2 e^{-K_2 t} + A_3 e^{-K_3 t} \quad (K_1 > K_2 > K_3) \quad (8.4)$$

where
A = an empirical constant
$K \, (= 0.693/t_{1/2})$ = the respective rate constant

The AUC in this case equals

$$AUC = \frac{A_1}{K_1} + \frac{A_2}{K_2} + \frac{A_3}{K_3} \tag{8.5}$$

In the above equation, A_3/K_3 represents the portion of the total AUC due to the terminal half-life. Example 2 illustrates the application of the above procedure.

Example 2

The intravenous administration of drugs A and B resulted in blood levels described by the following equations:

Drug A: $C = 447e^{-0.87t} + 57e^{-0.099t} + 29e^{-0.019t}$

Drug B: $C = 114e^{-0.41t} + 552e^{-0.042t} + 27e^{-0.011t}$

The area under curve values for the two drugs are calculated as follows:

Drug	A_1/K_1	A_2/K_2	A_3/K_3	AUC
A	514 (20%)[a]	576 (22%)	1526 (58%)	2616
B	278 (2%)	13143 (83%)	2455 (15%)	15876

[a]Parentheses indicate percent of total AUC.

For drug A, 58% of the AUC relates to the longest ("terminal") half-life whereas for drug B, only 15% of the AUC is due to the longest half-life. Thus, by ignoring the longest half-life, the value of AUC for drug A would be underestimated by 58% while that for drug B would be underestimated by 15% (Fig. 8.10). Since AUC is directly related to the predicted steady-state level (C_{ss}) as follows:

$$C_{ss} = \text{Dosing Rate} \times \text{AUC}/\text{Dose}_{iv} \tag{8.6}$$

it is apparent that the 36 hour half-life for drug A has a greater influence on C_{ss} than the substantially longer, 63 hour half-life for drug B.

Clearly, a long half-life only becomes important in dosing considerations when it contributes substantially to drug accumulation. The above method of estimating the relevance of a half-life, however, is only appropriate when a single component, i.e., unchanged drug or a metabolite, is measured, and should not be applied to evaluating total radioactivity profiles which include all drug-derived materials (parent drug plus metabolites). In a ra-

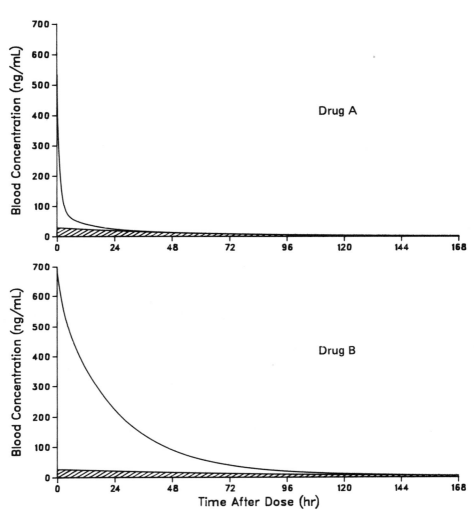

FIG. 8.10 The terminal half-life of drug A (36 hr) has a greater contribution to total AUC than that of drug B (63 hr).

dioactivity concentration versus time curve, the terminal phase usually represents a single component, i.e., the metabolite with the longest half-life, whereas the earlier phases of the curve often are composed of multiple entities (see Fig. 8.2). As stated previously, only under the rare circumstance when all metabolites as well as the parent drug have similar distribution volumes can the various AUC segments of the total radioactivity blood profile be compared. Consequently, in order to assess the relevance of the half-life obtained from a single dose in predicting radioactivity accumulation and the time required to reach steady state, multiple dosing experiments are recommended.

When a drug is repeatedly administered until steady state is achieved, the degree of accumulation can be estimated by one of the following equations:

$$R = \frac{AUC_{0-\tau(ss)}}{AUC_{0-\tau(1)}} \tag{8.7}$$

$$R = \frac{C_{min(ss)}}{C_{min(1)}} \tag{8.8}$$

where

R = the accumulation ratio

$AUC_{0-\tau(1)}$ and $AUC_{0-\tau(ss)}$ = the AUC values during a dose interval following a single dose and at steady state, respectively

$C_{min(1)}$ and $C_{min(ss)}$ = the blood concentrations immediately prior to the administration of the second dose and any dose at steady state, respectively

As shown in Fig. 8.11, the two methods should yield identical results. However, equation 8.7 is preferred if sufficient serial blood samples are

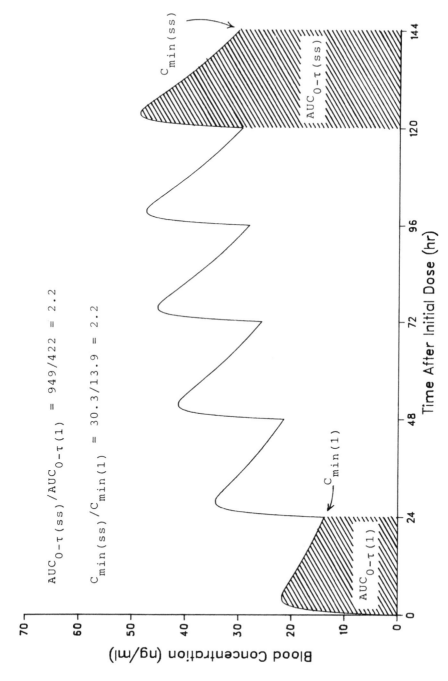

FIG. 8.11 Two methods of calculating the accumulation ratio using multiple-dose data.

available after dosing on both day 1 and at steady state to determine the respective AUC values. Equation 8.8 is more susceptible to error in that excessive weight is placed on a single determinant $C_{min(1)}$, even though $C_{min(ss)}$ can usually be obtained as the mean of several predose concentrations at steady state.

After determining the accumulation ratio, an effective half-life, i.e., one that is consistent with the observed accumulation of drug during chronic dosing, can be calculated as follows:

$$t_{1/2,\text{eff}} = \frac{0.693}{\omega}$$

where

$$\omega = -\frac{\ln(1 - 1/R)}{\tau}$$

The effective half-life is then compared with the half-life obtained from a single dose study to determine if the latter is relevant in predicting steady-state blood levels.

References

1. M. Gibaldi and D. Perrier, *Pharmacokinetics*, 2nd Ed., Marcel Dekker, New York, 1982, pp. 445-449.

2. P. G. Welling, *Pharmacokinetics: Processes and Mathematics*, American Chemical Society, Washington, D.C., 1986, pp. 193-195.

3. L. Z. Benet, Pharmacokinetic parameters: Which are necessary to define a drug substance? *Eur. J. Respir. Dis. (Suppl.)*, *65*:45-61, 1984.

Appendixes I-V

APPENDIX I Common Terminology Used in Drug Disposition Studies

Absolute bioavailability	The bioavailability of a dosage form relative to an intravenous dose.
Absorption	The process by which a compound and its metabolites are transferred from the site of absorption to the blood circulation.
Accumulation	The progressive increase of drug and/or metabolites in the body. Accumulation is influenced by the dosing interval and half-life of the drug. The process can be characterized by an "accumulation factor," which is the ratio of the plasma concentration at steady state to that following the first dose in a multiple dosing regimen.
Area under curve	The concentration of drug and/or metabolites in blood (or plasma/serum) integrated over time.
Bioavailability	The rate and extent to which a drug enters the systemic circulation intact. It is sometimes expanded to include therapeutically active metabolites.
Bioequivalence	A drug product is bioequivalent if its bioavailability is not significantly different, within a stated guideline, from that of a standard when administered at the same molar dose level.
Biopharmaceutics	The study of the pharmaceutical factors influencing bioavailability and the use of this information to control pharmacologic or therapeutic activity.
Biotransformation	The process by which the administered compound is structurally and/or chemically changed in the body by either enzymatic or non-enzymatic reactions. The product of the reaction is a different composition of matter or different configuration than the administered compound.
Clearance	The volume of biological fluid which is totally cleared of drug in a unit time.

Disposition	All processes and factors which are involved from the time a drug is administered to the time when it is eliminated from the body, either intact or in metabolite form.
Distribution	The process by which absorbed compound and/or its metabolites partition between blood and various tissues/organs in the body.
Dosage form	The gross pharmaceutical form (tablet, capsule, solution, etc.) administered to animals or man.
Dose proportionality	The relationship between doses of a drug and measured parameters, usually including tests for linearity.
Drug product	The finished dosage form, e.g., tablet, capsule, solution, suspension, that contains the active ingredient usually, but not necessarily, in association with inactive ingredients.
Enterohepatic circulation	The process by which drugs are emptied via the bile into the small intestine and then reabsorbed into the hepatic circulation.
Enzyme induction	The increase in enzyme content (activity and/or amount) due to xenobiotic challenge, which may result in more rapid metabolism of a compound.
Enzyme inhibition	The decrease in enzymatic activity due to the effect of xenobiotic challenge.
Excretion	The process by which the administered compound and/or its biotransformation product(s) are eliminated from the body.
First-order kinetics	Kinetic processes, the rate of which is proportional to the concentration.
First-pass effect	The phenomenon whereby drugs may be extracted or metabolized following enteral absorption before reaching the systemic circulation.

Half-life	The time elapsed for a given drug concentration or amount to change by a factor of two.
Hepatic clearance	The rate of total body clearance accounted for by the liver.
Lag time	The interval between drug administration and when the drug concentration is measurable in blood.
Metabolite characterization	The determination of physicochemical characteristics of the biotransformation product(s).
Metabolite identification	The structural elucidation of the biotransformation product(s).
Metabolite profile	The chromatographic pattern and/or aqueous/nonaqueous partitioning of the biotransformation products of the administered compound.
Nonlinear kinetics (saturation kinetics)	Kinetic processes, the rate of which is not directly proportional to the concentration.
Pharmacokinetics	The study of the kinetics of absorption, distribution, metabolism, and excretion of drugs.
Presystemic elimination	The loss of that portion of the dose that is not bioavailable. This would include, among others, loss through intestinal and gut-wall metabolism, lack of absorption, and first-pass hepatic metabolism.
Protein binding	The complexation of a drug and/or its metabolite(s) with plasma or tissue proteins.
Relative bioavailability	The bioavailability relative to a reference or standard dosage form.
Renal clearance	The rate of total body clearance accounted for by the kidney. Its magnitude is determined by the net effects of glomerular filtration, tubular secretion and reabsorption, renal blood flow, and protein binding.

Steady state	An equilibrium state where the rate of drug input is equal to the rate of elimination during a given dose interval.
Total clearance	The volume of biological fluid totally cleared of drug per unit time and usually includes hepatic clearance and renal clearance.
Volume of distribution	A hypothetical volume of body fluid into which the drug distributes. It is not a "real" volume, but is a proportionality constant relating the amount of drug in the body to the measured concentration in blood or plasma.

APPENDIX II   Life Span and Typical Body Weight of Selected Laboratory Animals

		Rat	Mouse	Dog[a]	Rabbit	Monkey[b]
Life span (yr)		2-3	3-3.5	10-14	5-7	20-30
Weight at birth (g)						
	M	6	1.5	240	50	475
	F	6	1.5	240	46	475
Adult weight (g)						
	M	250-500	20-25	8000-15000	1500-5000	3500-7500
	F	200-350	18-23	6000-12000	1500-5000	3500-6000

[a]Beagle
[b]Rhesus

APPENDIX III Typical Organ Weights in Adult Laboratory Animals

Organ	Percent of body weight				
	Rat	Mouse	Dog	Rabbit	Monkey
Liver	3.5	6	3.5	3	2.5
Kidney	0.8	1.6	0.5	0.8	0.5
Heart	0.4	0.4	0.8	0.3	0.4
Spleen	0.3	0.5	0.3	0.04	0.1
Brain	0.5	–	0.8	0.4	3
Adrenals	0.02	–	0.01	0.02	0.03
Lung	0.6	0.6	1	0.6	0.7

APPENDIX IV Approximate Volumes of Pertinent Biological Fluids in Adult Laboratory Animals

Fluid	Rat	Mouse	Dog	Rabbit	Monkey
Blood (ml/kg)	75	75	70	60	75
Plasma (ml/kg)	40	45	40	30	45
Urine (ml/kg/day)	60	50	30	60	75
Bile (ml/kg/day)	90	100	12	120	25

APPENDIX V   Reproduction Characteristics of the Mouse, Rat, and Rabbit

	Mouse	Rat	Rabbit
Age at mating (weeks)	6-10	9-14	24-35
Length of cycle (days)	4-5	4-5	–
Ovulation	Spontaneous	Spontaneous	Induced 10-11 hr postcoitus
Detection of mating	Vaginal plug, or sperm in smear	Vaginal plug, or sperm in smear	Copulation
Gestation period (days)	19-21	20-23	28-34
Litter size	6-12	6-15	5-10

Index